T0196493

ECT AND THE ELDERLY: SHOCKED FOR THE AGED

DEBORAH Y. LIGGAN, MD

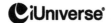

ECT AND THE ELDERLY:
SHOCKED FOR THE AGED

iUniverse books may be ordered through booksellers or by contacting:

iUniverse
1663 Liberty Drive
Bloomington, IN 47403
www.iuniverse.com
1-800-Authors (1-800-288-4677)

Because of the dynamic nature of the Internet, any web addresses or links contained in this book may have changed since publication and may no longer be valid. The views expressed in this work are solely those of the author and do not necessarily reflect the views of the publisher, and the publisher hereby disclaims any responsibility for them.

Any people depicted in stock imagery provided by Thinkstock are models, and such images are being used for illustrative purposes only. Certain stock imagery © Thinkstock.

ISBN: 978-1-5320-1714-8 (sc)
ISBN: 978-1-5320-1715-5 (e)

Library of Congress Control Number: 2017906785

Print information available on the last page.

iUniverse rev. date: 05/12/2017

Maintenance ECT

Bipolar disorder is expressed in emotional
      reactivity associated with loss in
      three-week cyclic suicide ideations.

As voices command me to contemplate
      my overdosing medications, or slitting my wrists,
      or hanging from a shower faucet.

Suicide is such a reality that I ask forgiveness
      for what I am about to do.

Voices reaffirm that I will only gain God's favor if I kill myself.

I acknowledge treatment for severe endogenous
      depression with each treatment I am destitute,
      And a fatal lease on life leaves me,
      Hoping that I am overwhelmed with the end of life.

I am aware at 9:00 am when I am transported
      to the Operating Room prep area,
      where I am pre-medicated with a muscle relaxant.
Then anesthetized by IV injection of a short acting barbiturate.

An electrode is placed over each temple
>and an alternating current of about
>400mA and 70 to 120V is passed
>between them for 0.1 to 0.5 seconds.

What is wrong with me?
>I contemplate victory as a life
>drains from my body and hope
>that death becomes a reality with each procedure.

When I awaken it is as if I am a new person of life.
>I will continue taking my medications
>to maintain steady moods during intervals
>between three-week maintenance treatments.

Deborah Y. Liggan, M.D.

Preface

There was a perceived need for a comprehensive study of geriatric ECT. Three questions must be answered when treating a patient with ECT:

1. Does the patient have an ECT-responsiveness illness?
2. Does the patient have any medical problems that might require modifications of technique or increase the risks of the procedure?
3. Has appropriate informed consent been obtained?

I agreed to use shock in the title because that is the name by which most people recognize the treatment. Modern ECT has come a long way since the 1930's origins (chapter one). In chapter four oxygenation, anesthesia, muscle relaxation, modifications in the form and doses of the energies, and variations in electrode placements have reduced the immediate cognitive effects, making the treatments more tolerable. Patients are fully anesthetized and relaxed during each induction. In addition, the consent process recognizes the importance of giving ECT to competent patients who consent voluntarily.

This book is written for those faced with decisions about the use of ECT and is meant to educate elderly patients about what they can expect. It is also meant to help students, medical practitioners, and mental health workers to intelligently identify and prepare elderly patients for treatment. My personal narrative in chapter six shares my experience with ECT. Four-teen years ago, I went through the first of five terrifying acute bipolar depressive episodes the changed my life forever. My first acute depression was the worse one in that I had no warning. And to make matters worse, all the medication trials that were prescribed to me were useless.

On two occasions I attempted suicide, resulting in ECT treatment. Over the next ten years, I relapsed into acute bipolar episodes four more times. But I was prepared. I knew what worked for me, so I wasted no time in getting ECT treatments. Between psychotic depressive episodes, I went back to school to get a medical degree. This qualified me to author multiple medical articles and a medical textbook targeting African American elderly. My second book, The Veteran's Guide to Psychiatry, played a central role in the provision of mental health services that impact on the veteran's life. Readers who are interested in learning more about the research conducted on ECT can consult the publications listed in the Bibliography.

Acknowledgements

This book is the product of more than 15 years of interest in electroshock. A number of geriatric patients gave generously of their time in interviews, especially working as monitor of my condition. In the interests of accuracy, I tried to interview as many people involved with my life, my illness and my treatments as possible.

I would like to acknowledge the many people in my life journey that I consider blessed by their presence. I also thank the nurses and aides who were responsible for the daily care of these patients; without their support and faith, the clinical studies drawn upon here would not have been possible. Each person was involved by giving the manuscript in a critical reading to tell the story from my own point of view.

I have been very fortunate in the course of writing this book to have had the help and support of many wonderful people along the way. First and foremost, my two amazing children, Desiree and Rachael-their understanding, encouragement, love and support story provided the courage I needed to forge ahead with this project. To my typist Desiree Fawn Liggan, I would like to give special thanks for the typing and word processing of many drafts and for her encouragement through our publication.

This book owes a special debt to my parents, Moses and Alberta Brooks, who encouraged me to tackle the subject, which I conceived as a study of geriatric electro-convulsive therapy. As it became apparent that telling the ECT story involved by giving the manuscript a critical reading to tell the story from my own pint of view.

Corliss Clayton, a soul sister, who believed in my ability way before I believed in myself. Her relentless spirit and passion fueled my own spirit and passion to finally finish this book.

And finally, my utmost gratitude to the many health care professionals at the Psychosocial Rehabilitation and Recovery Center (PRRC) whose care I depended on in my darkest moments.

Thank you

List of Tables and Figure

Contents

Chapter One

The History of ECT

The ancient Greeks were the first to dream of an electric cure. They believed there were special curative powers in the seizures of epileptics. This was followed by the early Romans who put those powers to the rest by treating head pain by generating an electric pulse potent enough to produce a convulsion.

The theory was: the more severe the convulsion, the better the results. According to the primitive technology two electrodes were strapped to the patient's head, then, at a nod from the doctor, a nurse plugged the other end of the cord directly into the wall outlet. There was no shock machine to control the safety of the current or its duration. At a second sign from the doctor, the nurse unplugged the cord, the patient had a seizure, and all was presumed to be well. Those early patients often let out a shriek as the electricity was applied, but as they convulsed they blacked out.

1.1 Convulsive Therapy

Electroconvulsive therapy (ECT) was introduced in the 1930's at a time when no effective treatment for the severe mentally ill was

1

known. Convulsive therapy, in the form of chemically induced seizures, was first tested in the 1930's in patients with dementia praecox, a disorder that is now widely labeled as schizophrenia (Meduna 1935, 1937; Fink 1979).

The induction of a seizure by Metrazol was a frightening procedure. Within a few minutes after the intravenous injection, the patient's thoughts began to race, his heart beat more rapidly, he experienced feelings of terror and impending doom, and suddenly lost consciousness. When he awakened, his muscles and back ached, often his tongue and lips were bleeding, and he had a violent headache.

A successful method was designed in Rome by Ugo Cerletti and Lucio Bini, where a seizure was safely induced electrically. The original Cerletti method relied on alternating current from a wall socket the pulsed from positive to negative at forty-five cycles per second (45 hertz). This form of current is calling a "sine wave".

Just how fast shock was catching on became clear in a U.S. Public Health Service Survey in October 1941, barely eighteen months after the treatment arrived in America. At this time physicians were already experimenting with drugs to relax the muscles and reduce fractures and dislocations.

1.2 Fink's Introduction of ECT

Dr. Max Fink was first and foremost among clinicians introducing ECT. He watched his first ECT as a medical student in the 1940's and started giving it regularly during his residency in 1952, ECT's heyday. Electroconvulsive Therapy (ECT) has been used for nearly seventy years to treat mental illness. As ECT pioneer Max Fink puts it: except for penicillin for neuro-syphilis and niacin for pellagra, ECT for severe illness is the most effective treatment developed in the twentieth century. So clear are the benefits of ECT for patients who might otherwise commit suicide, or languish for years in the blackness of depression, that there should be little controversy over whether it is safe or effective. The assertion that ECT is associated with memory loss, but in the vast majority of patients, memory is restored within weeks after the last treatment, suggesting that no long-term damage to the brain's memory capacities is sustained. In addition, it was used for the treatment of the deep sadness of melancholia, the delusion of psychotic depression, the unceasing restlessness of mania, or the hallucination of schizophrenia. ECT proved again and again that it was too valuable to be jettisoned with its sister therapies. It survived because it was needed and it worked.

By the mid 1950's, patients were getting high doses of oxygen along with their anesthesia and muscle relaxant (Falk and Zangerl, 2005). What Fink described were some of first efforts to map the effects of both psychotropic drugs and ECT on the electroencephalograph (EEG), which is a quantitative surface recording of overall patterns of brain activity. Monitoring ECT treatments with an EEG was encouraged; this was to make sure that a proper grand mal seizure had occurred. Ironically, this is what Cerletti believed in the 1940's; it took a full sixty years for the rest of the medical community to agree.

The current view is that efficacy and amnesia are unrelated. In 1979, Max Fink wrote in his guide to ECT: "the elimination of amnesia should not interfere with therapeutic efficacy." The patients were first given an intravenous injection rapidly. When the maximum effect was apparent after about 80 seconds, the shock was given, along with oxygen. When it was evident that the patient's breathing was regular and that there was a free airway, he was returned to the ward. It was described in the practice of ECT what was later judged a brutal spectacle of uncontrollable thrashing to a calm scene in which scarcely a muscle moved, the clinicians' only clue to a cerebral seizure taking place being the twitching of the patient's big toe, a blood pressure cuff having been wrapped about the calf to ensure that the succinylcholine would not reach the muscles that control the toe, so the evidence of a fit would be visible.

ECT survived the excess of its golden age in the 1940's, 1950's and 1960's. With the psychologist's professional bias toward talk therapy and against trying to shock patients out of their anguish. In the 1980's, it was an era when shock doctors were likened to Spanish inquisitors and ECT because the bete noire of film and books. Psychiatrists not only enjoyed the movie <u>One Flew Over the Cuckoo's Nest</u> enough to see it twice, followed by agreement with its premise that patients have too little clout and organized psychiatry that has more than its merits.

With the advancement of Jan-Otto Ottosson's theory that the seizure itself was the therapeutic agent in ECT, clinicians suggested that excess electrical current was responsible for memory problems. This led during the 1970's and 1980's to a widespread replacement of the sine wave machine with an apparatus capable of delivering brief pulses of treatment.

A leading ECT critic, Dr. John Friedberg, was right that there were studies pointing to neurological changes in the beginning, when electroshock was given without oxygen to protect the brain, more treatments were given at higher intensity, and damage was more likely and less of a concern to psychiatrists and patients desperate for an effective treatment. In 1984, Dr. Richard Weiner of Duke University undertook a review of the ECT literature similar to Friedberg's nearly a decade earlier (1991). How well does ECT work for its target population of severely depressed patients? Doctors have been drawn to electroshock for a single reason: it helped when no other treatment did, not even wonder drugs. That doesn't mean jumping to ECT immediately, of course. But it does mean instituting some kind of effective treatment quickly and vigorously. This is how psychiatry saw how ECT could help people who did not respond to anything else. Treatments were administered for major depressive disorder, particularly the psychotic form malignant catatonia in carious form; phase's labeled acute schizophrenia; and manic disorder (Abrams 2002; APA 2001; and Fink 1999). Considered also, Parkinson's disease and neuroleptic malignant syndrome are two their medical conditions where ECT is used, sometimes with remarkable effect.

Table 1-1. Common Medical Conditions in which ECT was used to treat patients with remarkable effect:

- Chronic Obstructive pulmonary Disease (COPD)
- Asthma
- Hypertension
- Coronary Artery Disease
- History of Myocardial Infarction
- Cardiac Arrhythmia
- History of Cerebrovascular accident
- Osteoporosis

A greater alliance between psychiatrists and anesthesiologists has encouraged treatment teams competent to manage the most severe medically ill patient for whom ECT is a life-saving consideration (Abrams 1989). And just as the trifecta of anesthesia, muscle relaxant, and oxygen had helped overcome the treatment's bone-breaking image in the 1950's, so thirty years later electroshock was crossing an equally momentous threshold scientific precision that made it more attractive for doctors to give it to patients.

If it were up to Dr. Leon Rosenberg, who credits ECT with restoring his health if not just saving his lie, the procedure would be acailable to all pateints and used sooner by more of them Ther is little doubt that ECT will be used more widely in the future that it is now. It simply too beneficial to be used as a last resort.

1.3 The Golden Era of ECT

The most honest appraisal for the state of knowledge about ECT during tis golden era came from California's Department of Mental Hygiene, which noted in the 1950-52 Biennial Report that "the exact mechanism by which electroshock therapy helps unscramble twisted emotions and thought processes is something no one understands completely even after years of continuing research." What is key is that ECT releases chemicals to make the brain cells work better, althoguhprecisely own that happens is open to dueling theories.

In days of Jim Crow Laws and systematic segregation of African Amereicans, Cnetral State Hosptial in Petersburg, Virginia, served exclusively black patients. Conditions ther were so deadly that it was a public embarrassment to the state. In 1955, Judge Hoffman considered a lawsuit arising out of care at Central, stating "Virginia has completely failed in its obligations to the mentally ill, both white and colored." Other than electric shock treatments occasionally administerd, there is not treatment afforded to the patients. They eat, sleep, and sit—this is the routine day. If the shock treatments do not bring favorable results, the patients wait to die. In the 1950's, so thirty years later electroshock was crossing an equally momentous threshold scientific precision that made it more attractive for doctors to give to patients.

Under the influence of Harold Sackeim, a professor of psychiatry at Columbia Psychiatric Institute, it became the norm to limit the amount of electricity used to dose only marginally in excess of the seizure threshold. His first publication on ECT was in 1983, and in 1985 he joined the editorial board of the Journal of ECT (Convulsive Therapy).

1.4 Outpatient ECT

ECT does not require admission to a hospital. It can be done safely and effectively on an outpatient basis, and in the years form 1938 to about 1970, a majority of treatments took place in the offices of psychiatrists, neurologists, and family doctors, rather than in mental hospitals. Most commonly, it was for maintenance treatment, giving it on Saturday morning so that the patient could continue to hold a job and not have to enter a mental hospital.

In 1949 William Karliner began publishing his techniques, and his papers form the early 1950's were widely read as practical guides for outpatients ECT. The treatment by academic psychiatrists often spoke scornfully of him because he saw so many patients. Yet over the years his patients experienced few side effects. He had only one death in almost fifty years of practice: and there is no doubt that he made life more tolerable for many families with afflicted relatives who preferred the outpatient clinic to the hospital ward.

ECT specialists during this era tried hard to reduce memory impairment by decreasing the amount of electricity flowing into the brain while at the same time producing an effective seizure. It was believed that there was a trade-off between memory loss and therapeutic efficacy: the less effect on memory, the less efficacious the treatment of the illness itself.

In 1953, the American Psychiatric Association ratified the legitimacy of outpatient ECT. Patients were selected who were in good health who may be treated as ambulatory, provided that the therapist took special precautions in using intravenous sedation or a muscle relaxant such as curare. This process took place before the introduction of reliable muscle relaxants (which curare was not), oxygen supplementation, and a short-acitng barbiturate anesthetic. In 1951, the problem of fractures was solved with the introduction of succinylcholine.

1.5 Self-Assessment Questions

1. In what way did the early Romans treat head pain by using electricity?

2. Describe the use of electricity based on the theory that was the more severe the convulsion, the better the results.

3. What disorders were used to treat convulsive therapy in the form of chemically induced seizures?

4. Describe the form of current based on a "sine wave" designed by Cerletti and Bini.

5. What doctor was first to describe the effects of both psychotropic drugs and ECT on the electroencephalograph (EEG) to record brain activity?

6. What is the key that makes ECT release chemicals that make brain cells work better?

7. How is impedance variable between individual patients receiving ECT?

8. In what medical conditions was ECT used to treat with remarkable effect?

9. Describe the great alliance between psychiatrists and anesthesiologists.

10. What doctor established the norm to limit the amount of electricity used to dose only marginally in excess of the seizure threshold?

Chapter Two

Madness Cured with Electricity

How do seizures, which can be dangerous and damaging when they occur spontaneously, change a dysfunctional brain into one that performs normally?

Table 2-1. Psychoanalysis and ECT:

- It must be said that not all psychoanalysts were hostile to the administration of ECT.
- Most analysts did not keep records of their ECT patients.
- Using Freud as their model, analysts looked for circumstances unknown to the patient and submerged in the unconscious realm.
- At a basic level, the analyst were unable to accept that a jolt of electricity lasting one-fifth of a second that it might achieve a better result than months of drawn-out talk therapy.
- For the schizophrenic and melancholic patients receiving convulsive therapy neither was nor part of the elective terrain of psychoanalysis.
- Despite all the vitriolic fervor in public discourse, ECT was the secret love of psychoanalysis.

- It was that the whole biological logic of the shock therapies starkly contradicted the psychogenic thinking of psychoanalysis.
- The main objection to convulsion therapy is that it comes as an escape from the acceptance of the psychology of the unconscious.
- It was much healthier to compel patients to cope with their unconscious minds in psychotherapy sessions than to lift symptoms with ECT mechanical procedures.
- Anything other than stark, raving madness belongs on the couch, not the treatment table.
- Psychoanalysis and ECT flowed smoothly back and forth, with world-famous analysts offering psychoanalytic formulations of their problems.
- Researchers did extensive work on shock therapies, investigating barbiturate anesthetics, looking at ketogenic diets in ECT, and studying the effect of shock treatments on memory.

2.1 Shock Therapy

The ECT story began with shock therapy, which is a method for treating certain mental or emotional conditions by stimulating the brain electrically in order to produce a cerebral seizure. In medicine, the term shock implies hypothermia (low body temperature) and hypotension (low blood pressure). It can occur during exposure to harsh weather conditions, particularly when the body is both wet and cold, or surgically as a result of blood loss. So shock has long been a familiar medical concept because anaphylactic shock is caused by a sudden discharge of histamine in an allergic reaction. Injecting various substances to modify the action of the autonomic nervous system; to raise or lower vascular tone or body temperature; or to stimulate the action of the bowels. In some asylums, infected teeth were rooted out on the grounds that they might cause autointoxication, a kind of systemic poisoning that might involve the brain itself. In addition, there was a vogue for colectomy, removing part of the large bowel on the grounds that toxins leading from the gut might instigate madness. Deep sleep therapies, using barbiturates to make patients stuporous for weeks on end, gained wide currency. Its significance laid in the fact that it acts more quickly than drugs and is better tolerated by patients, who faced the feeling of dread they experienced with the drug as the loss of consciousness loomed. Knowing what makes ECT effective also would help with a series of more targeted techniques researchers who test to stimulate the brain without the need for full-fledged seizures and with for fewer side effects.

In 1926, the Parisian psychiatrist constance Pascal introduced the word shock to psychiatry. As a young medical graduate of Romanian origin, she had been in 1908 the first female psychiatrist in France to join the elite Parisian asylum Psychiatrists. In her 1926 book on "shock treatment, "she deplored the previous therapeutic nihilism of psychiatry: "To have to look on helplessly at the fatal advance of psychosis, to indifferently note demented immobility and the transition ot endorse fate; accepting the predisposition to delusions and the fatal destiny of constitution also means renouncing the practical application of the biological sciences that have modified the study of general pathology." Pascal argued that mental illness originated for "mental anaphylactic reactions." To combat it, one needed to shock the brain and the autonomic nervous system back into equilibrium. This shock should be capable of preventing, of suspending or of curing these mental ananphylactic manifestations. She argued that the body ight be shocked by the injection of various substances such as colloidal gold, milk, or vaccines, or by the kind of fecer therapy that Julius Wagner-Jauregg had just introduced in Vienna against neurosyphilis. Today she is virtually unknown, and after World

War II her enthusiasm for these peculiar injections was seen as horrific. Though Pascal brought the concept of shock to psychiatry, she did not mean it in the ense of convulsions, which she as at pains to avoid with her various therapies.

Electroconvulsive therapy, in which brain seizures are induced, is not the same as electric shock, which refers to a form of psychological therapy in which shocks are delivered to induce pain so that subjects will refrain from performing an unwanted behavior. At one time, this practice was used to stop the self-injurious behaviors of scratching, head banging, and screaming of intellectually disabled patients. Electrical energy is characterized by an alternate experimental. An alternate experimental method that was developed by psychologists; to approximate the seizure threshold. During the first treatment an electrical stimulus is applied, beginning with the first, which is too low and increased until a seizure is produced. Successive treatments are given with energy doses that are a fixed amount above the estimate threshold.

Basing their views on Freudian theory, researchers imagined that seizures suppressed memories of childhood trauma that they deemed to be the basis for psychological symptoms (Janis, 1950). Max Fink (2009) reports that elderly patients are often considered for ECT, especially when they also suffers from a systemic illness or do not tolerate their medications. They may be depressed and threaten suicide, refuse food and fluids, be so overactive that they risk exhaustion and self-injury, threaten to harm themselves or others, or be in a melancholic stupor.

2.2 Insulin Coma Therapy

ECT is a procedure, in which, an electric current is applied across scalp electrodes to induce a grand mal seizure. The procedure was introduced in 1938 in Italy by Ugo Cerlett and Lucio Bini to replace less reliable convulsive therapies that used liquid chemicals. ECT us one of the oldest medical treatments still in regular use, a fact that attests to its safety and efficacy. Its mechanism of action remains a mystery, yet it is known to produce multiple effects on the CNS, including the down regulation of B-receptors, a property that ECT has in common with most an ti-depressants. That is why the anticonvulsant theory suggests that the anti-depressant effect of ECT is related to the fact that ECT itself exerts a profound anticonvulsant effect on the brain.

Where Sackheim and George focused on stimulating specific circuits, Fink and others argued that seizures are necessary and that these probably act through the release or inhibition of some endocrine factor, such as cortisol. After Cerletti and Bini's presentation at the Academy of Medicine, news spread quickly about an effective new treatment for schizophrenia. Families of patients from all over Italy wrote to the clinic, and patients treated with electric jolts began to her better. "Madness cured with electricity" was the headline of this story. Even Cerletti hoped to isolate a hormone changed by ECT, which could be given instead of the electrical shocks. At the University of Budapest psychiatry clinic somatotherapies for schizophrenia had been under way since World War I. Clinics were experimented with giving large doses on insulin, and in 1928 Julius Schuster (who had earlier published results on inducing anaphylactic shock) proposed treating psychosis with shock and insulin together. By the late 1920's various researchers came across the idea of deliberately putting psychiatric patients into hypoglycemic insulin comas. In 1929, the mental hospital in Lausanne-Cery, the psychiatrist Hans Steck was responsible for the hypoglycemic treatment of psychosis, though he was careful to avoid producing overly deep comas and convulsion. Steck and French medical journals, and his work was not widely known. In those days insulin was often mentioned in the medical press. It was discovered in 1922 at the

University of Toronto as the chemical governing the uptake of sugar from the blood stream and employed in the treatment of diabetes. But it was soon used to treat nondiabetic illness as well. In psychiatric clinics it was mainly given to undernourished patients to encourage appetite. At the University of Vienna psychiatry clinic gave insulin to a number of patients with delirium tremens, a term used to describe the psychosis and shakes of withdrawal from alcohol.

It is documented in the medical literature that Manfred Sakel was the attending psychiatrist, and he and his colleagues at the clinics diagnosed the patient with schizophrenia. On the day following his admission, Sakel injected the patient with 45 units of insulin. Nothing happened. That evening the patient was still praranoid and hallucinotic, and refused his dinner, claiming it was poisoned. The next morning he was given three injections of 40 units of insulin each. He became calmer. At noon he was given injection of 50 units and went to hypoglycemic shock. Insulin causes the liver and muscles to remove circulating glucose from the brain blood, which means denying it as well to the brain. In the absence of glucose the brain goes into a coma or a stupor, which is called, "insulin shock". When this patient awakened spontaneously from the coma; he was rational and apologized for all the trouble that he had caused. But then his condition worsened again. In the third week of treatment with insulin injection, with no warning signs, the patient experienced a major attack of epilepsy one and a half hours after an injection of 50 units of insulin, displaying tonic-clonic convulsions (muscles flexing and extending) and biting his tongue. After the seizure, the patient had complete amnesia for the preceding events and his memory loss lasted an hour and a half. But as it returned, including recall of the beginning of the convulsion, he had complete insight into the pathological nature of his previous behavior. From his clinical notes on this first patient, it is clear that Sakel was not trying to induce a seizure, for the patient's sudden convulsion took him and his assistant off guard. That the patient bit his tongue indicated they had no time to insert a mouth block and this failed to anticipate the convulsive effect. In 1950, Sakel told the Paris World Psychiatry Congress that he had initially conceived his procedure as a convulsive therapy but then realized that convulsions were damaging to the brain, making the illness worse, and that the procedure was in fact a coma therapy (Coma and Seizures are both forms of shock). Still later, as Sakel realized that electroconvulsive therapy was the wave of the future and insulin coma therapy was being widely abandoned, he had yet another version that would let him claim paternity of the somatic treatments.

2.3 Metrazol Convulsion Therapy

This was superior to insulin coma therapy because it was safer-patients in deep coma were often at the brink of death. The insulin treatment had a death rate of 2 to 10 percent. The essential factor in Metrazol therapy was the convulsion, whereas in insulin coma the agent was hypoglycemia. Metazol's appeal in the United States was its efficacy in mood disorders. Depression was considered unresponsive to insulin, and the convention quickly grew up that insulin coma was to be reserved for what everyone was calling schizophrenia, and Metrazol should be used for affective disorders. By 1941, Metrazol had become even more popular than insulin in American mental hospitals.

2.4 The Neurotransmitter Theory

Dopamine is the neurotransmitter involved in motivation, emotional significance, relevance, focus, and pleasure. It helps the patient get things done. Foods that tend to increase dopamine include beef, poultry, fish, eggs, seeds (pumpkin and sesame), nuts (almonds and walnuts) cheese, protein powders, and green tea. Tyrosine is the amino acid building block for dopamine and is also essential for thyroid function. That is why simple carbohydrates tend to deplete dopamine.

Serotonin is a neurotransmitter that helps soothe the brain. It is intimately involved in sleep, mood regulation, appetite, and social engagement. It helps decrease worries and concerns. Foods rich in simple carbohydrates have been found to quickly boost serotonin. They cause a spike in insulin, which lowers most large amino acids with the exception of tryptophan, the amino acid building block for serotonin, thereby decreasing the competition for tryptophan to get into the brain. This is why many people can become dependent on or even addicted to bread, pasta, potatoes, rice, and sugar. They use these as "mood foods" and feel more relaxed and less worried after they eat them.

According to the neurotransmitter theory, ECT is known to enhance dopaminergic, serotonergic, and adrenergic neurotransmission. The fact that ECT has clear antiparkinsonian effects argues strongly for dopaminergic enhancement. That ECT also has profoundly anti-psychotic effects (and it is expected that decreases in dopamine function is associated with anti-psychotic affect (and it is expected that decreases in dopamine function is associated with anti-psychotic effects) argues against a single theory of increased dopamine availability throughout the brain. In addition, the serotonin system is the only monaminergic system in which ECT is believed to have opposite effects from most antidepressant drugs. The major metabolite of serotonin was increased in the spinal fluid of patients after ECT. Finally, the adrenergic system is affected by ECT.

2.5 Sources of Seizures

Coroboration of a grand mal seizure comes from three sources: an electrocardiogram that shows a spike in heart rate, an electroencephalogram that reveals changes in the brain's electrical activity, and a blood pressure cuff that reflects an increase in pressures. The whole routine, from the time a patient counts herself to sleep to when she is moved to the recovery bay, normally takes less than fifteen minutes and is often over in five.

Electroconvulsive therapy can be safely administered to most psychiatric patients. In the elderly, the risk is those related to physical deterioration associated with aging. ECT has been safely administered to patients as old as 102 although the list of systematic problems in the elderly is long, none prevents the use of ECT. Some conditions, however, make it more difficult to administer anesthetics and maintain good oxygenation. Therefore, elderly and systemically ill patients are treated in a hospital by skilled practitioners.

The films <u>One Flew over the Cuckoo's Nest and, A Beautiful Mind</u> portray Hollywood images of the treatment. It pictures the dramatic scene of a pleading patient dragged to a treatment room, forcibly administered electric currents as his jaw clenches, his back arches, and his body shakes while being held down by burly attendants or by foot and wrist restraints. The truth is that patients are not covered into treatment. They may be anxious and reluctant, but they come willingly. They have been told why the treatment is recommended, the procedures have been explained, and many have seen videos images of the procedures. The result is the application of the Hippocratic axiom "<u>premium non nocere</u>" (above all, do no harm), which combines the principles of beneficence and non-maleficence: "I will use treatment to help the sick according to my ability and judgment, but I will never use it to injure or wrong them."

The most vexing questions facing potential ECT patients and their families require that these questions be answered:

- Does the patient have an ECT responsive illness?
- At what point in the illness should ECT be explored?
- How often is treatment recommended?
- Does the patient have any medical problems that might require modifications of technique or increase the risks of the procedures?
- What technique should be used to set the dose of electricity?
- What is documented about memory loss and other possible side effects?
- Has appropriate informed consent been obtained?

Who are we to say who should risk experiencing the side effects of ECT rather than those of one medication or another? When it comes to effectiveness, ECT works more often, more quickly, and more thoroughly than any other treatment option available to those who suffer many brain illnesses. ECT starts working in one to two weeks, versus medication therapies that can take six to eight weeks. The faster that a treatment works, the sooner patients can start rebuilding their lives. Quick treatment can improve quality of life; halt the damage to diminish financial challenges. Patients experience less dementia, or cognition decline, than individuals with untreated brain illness. Depression, for example, is associated with an increased risk of subsequent dementia when untreated. Consider pharmacology augmenting ECT. As we age, medications metabolize differently, interact more, and can cause life threatening side effects. Even medication that a patient has taken safely for years can, one day out of the blue, cause dizziness and falls. It starts by causing nausea.

By the advent of the twenty first century, convulsive therapy passed from a highly stigmatized procedures obtained only in extreme circumstances to a helpful treatment available as a matter of course in many centers. The utility of ECT was not limited to psychiatric illnesses such as schizophrenia, depression, suicidal ideation, and mania. When a patient expresses a suicidal idea, it becomes absolutely imperative to proceed to ECT. The idea recedes after two or three treatments, even if the depression as such is not relieved. In later years, even Parkinsonism was treated with convulsive therapy.

2.6 Cerletti's Electrical Activity

The ECT story began shortly after Cerletti's arrival in Genoa. In line with his interest in tissue changes in the central nervous system. In 1931 he decided to determine whether the hippocampus (a region in the brain now known to play a role in lerning and memory) was involved in epilepsy. It was then suggested to him that electricity might be a nontoxic way of inducing epilepsy in dogs. To ensure that the tissue would not be changed by the convulsive agent itself, Cerletti placed one electrode in the animal's mouth and the other in the rectum-so as not to pass electricity directly through the brain itself.

However, the mortality of the procedure was very high because the current passed through the dog's heart, disrupting its electrical (pacemaker) activity.

When Cerletti was called to professorship in Rome, he wanted to continue his research and asked an assistant professor at the clinic, Lucio Bini, to help him with this work. Bini built a machine that could conveniently cause seizures in dogs with controlled doses of electricity. With the aid of the clinics electrician, he constructed a primitive machine that had a stopwatch for controlling the duration of current and a rheostat for adjusting the voltage. It was designed to use alternating current from wall sockets. Meanwhile, in 1935 Laszlo Meduna announced his finding that inducing fits with Metrazol could relieve schizophrenia. This news caused awareness in the Cerletti team that their electrical method of inducing seizures was applicable to schizophrenic treatment. The first step was to establish through animal research that electricity could be applied safely. Public images of electrocutions and capital punishment using an electric chair served to raise concerns, and the whole idea of applying electricity in convulsive doses seemed culturally ill-starred.

Until advent of the anti-depressant drugs, ECT was the treatment of choice for the agitated depression of middle and late life. The rate of ECT use in the Medicare population increased from 4.2 per 10,000 beneficiaries in 1987 to 5.1 in 1992. Between 20,000 and 35,000 suicides are recorded annually in the United States, and attempted suicides exceed this number by about 10 times. According to current statistics, suicide is the ninth leading cause of death in America, a figure that emphasizes the importance of recognizing depressions that have a high potential for self-destruction. Therefore, every physician should be familiar with the few clues that identify those patients who intend to end their lives.

The medical community poses the question, when doesn't ECT work? Ernest Hemingway suffered psychotic depression and committed suicide despite receiving ECT treatments. One must bear in mind that he was a chronic alcoholic. Therefore, alcoholics have a high seizure threshold and often are unresponsive to the ECT.

When is the treatment most successful? ECT does not require admission to a hospital. It can be done safely and effectively on an outpatient basis, and in the years from 1938 to about 1970, a majority of treatment took place in the offices of psychiatrist, neurologists, and family doctors, rather than in mental hospitals.

With anesthesia and barbiturate as part of the procedure, ECT now has to be done in a hospital. We are reminded that barbiturate anesthesia depresses a patient's respiratory centers (respiration is already interrupted for forty seconds or so by the shock itself) and entails the presence of an anesthetist, in case resuscitation is necessary.

What about side effects? When I talk about ECT, curious patients often ask me about possible brain damage. The truth is that ECT does not cause brain damage, change your personality, or turn you into Frankenstein's relative. It also does not affect metabolism, heart, weight, appetite, sex drive, sexual performance, cause dry mouth, vomiting, diarrhea, life-threatening rash, or any other common or bizarre side effects. Instead, studies show that the side effects of ECT are generally headaches and temporary memory loss.

2.7 Self-Assessment Questions

1. How does Freudian theory describe suppressed memories of childhood trauma?

2. What is the function of cortisol in the production of seizures?

3. What product of the serotonin system is the only monaminergic system in which ECT is believed to have opposite effects from most antidepressant drugs?

4. What three sources indicate corroboration of a grand mal seizure?

5. Define what is the result of the Hippocratic axiom "premium non nocere."

6. Describe the treatments of patients by Sakel with insulin injections producing hypoglycemic shock.

7. What is the efficiency of starting to work between medication or ECT?

8. According to medical statics, when doesn't ECT work?

9. What are the differences between Metrazol convulsion therapy and insuli coma therapy?

10. What do studies show that are the side effects of ECT?

Chapter Three

Patient Preparation

The goals of the pre-ECT evaluation are to 1) determine whether ECT is indicated, 2) establish baseline psychiatric and cognitive status to serve as a reference point for assessing patient response and cognitive side effects, 3) identify and treat any medical factors that may be associated with an increased risk of adverse effects from ECT, and 4) initiate the process of informed consent.

Table 3-1. Pre-ECT Evaluation

Medical and psychiatric history
Physical examination
Mental status examination
Laboratory evaluation (in selected cases)
       Electrocardiogram
       Complete blood count
       Electrolytes
       Liver function tests
       Other tests specific to patient's medical condition

Anesthesia Consultation

Consider (in selected cases)

>   Computed tomography or magnetic resonance imaging of the head
>
>   Electroencephalogram
>
>   Chest X-ray

3.1 Assessment of the Older Patient

The elderly patient presenting for diagnostic evaluation must be assessed carefully. Evaluation should include a thorough history of the presenting complaint, previous psychiatric illness, medical history, medication use, family history, social history, habits and use of alcohol, and a mental status examination including appearance, affect, behavior, mood, thought, and cognition. An essential element is the assessment of functional capacity, which aids in diagnosis as well as in treatment planning. Perhaps the most significant area in which the assessment of older patients differs from that of younger ones is in the evaluation of cognitive deficits.

Clinical signs and symptoms of disease in the older patient are often blunted, absent, or atypical. A good example is thyrotoxicosis. Compared with the younger patient, who typically presents with a variety of classic signs and symptoms such as nervousness, weight loss, tremor, and tachycardia. Elderly patients are more likely to present with cognitive dysfunction, anorexia, muscle weakness, atrial fibrillation, or congestive heart failure.

Often, only subtle and nonspecific signs and symptoms, such as a change in mental status, increased lethargy, a diminished appetite, or an increased frequency of falls, suggest that an underlying acute illness is present. Although psychiatric symptoms such as depressed mood, personality change, or inattentiveness may indicate the presence of infection, congestive heart failure, or a metabolic disorder, a true psychiatric problem such as depression may manifest with constitutional symptoms such as headache or weakness and dizziness.

3.2 The Mental Status Examination

A careful mental status examination is an essential tool in the evaluation of any patient with memory loss and should include the following assessments:

Sensorium or level of consciousness. This is usually described on a continuum which includes the terms alett, lethargic, drowsy, sleepy, stuporous, and comatose. Both the actual state of consciousness and the presence of fluctuations of consciousness should be noted. If the patient is anything but alert, delirium should be suspected.

Orientation. Ask the patient his name, date of birth where he is the season and exact date. Brain dysfunction as in delirium and dementia, usually produces a more marked and all-encompassing disorientation although this will vary with the severity of the illness.

Attention. Valid testing of memory requires that attention be relatively unimpaired. Have the patient repeat digits forward and backward. A normal elderly individual should be able to repeat six numbers forward and five backward. Another test of attention is to read out a series of letters or numbers and ask the patient to indicate, by tapping the desk, every time a particular letter or number is repeated. This skill is markedly impaired in delirium; less so in dementia and pseudo dementia. Attention should be normal in amnestic syndromes.

Memory. Short-term memory is tested by having the patient recall three or fur objects after 10 minutes. If the patien is unable to recall the wordsm the examiner can provide caregorical, phonemic, or contextual clues. Short-term memory is impaired in delirium, amnesia, dementia, and depressive pseudodementia. However, it is often not testable in delirium because of severe inattention.

Long-term memory is tested by asking the patient about verification past events, both personal and impersonal, such as the date of marriage, place of birth, details of work history, the names of past presidents, and dates of the world wars. List short-term memory, long-0term memory is often not testable in delirium because of inattention. Long-term memory becomes impaired in the middle and late phases or stages of dementia. In amnestic syndrome, long-term memory is less severely affected than short-term memory and it is usually intact in depressive pseudodementia.

Appearance. The patient's hygiene, grooming, and appropriateness of dress should be noted. In delirium and in moderate to severe dementia, patients are often disheveled but show little awareness or concern. Patients who are cognitively impaired secondary to depression will usually show deterioration in self-care of which they are aware but unmotivated to change. Dressing errors such as socks of different colors, articles of clothing put on backward, and buttons fastened incorrectly are usually reliable signs of organic disease. Patients suffering from and amnestic syndrome would not typically show deterioration in their appearance and hygiene.

Behavior. The examiner should observe the patient's manner of greeting and his or her general attitude toward the interview. Bewilderment, suspiciousness, or denial of the need to see a doctor are often noted in delirious and demented individuals. Gait disturbances, abnormal involuntary movements, and fluctuations in behavior are indications of bran disease and should be noted.

Affect and Mood. The patient's affect and mod state are important to assess. Does the patient appear depressed? How bothered is the patient by the memory impairment? A disturbance of affect and mood as well as complaints about memory disturbance are usually more prominent in patients with pseudodementia than in patients with delirium, amnestic syndrome and dementia who do not have a secondary psychiatric disturbance.

Thought Content. The examiner should inquire about the presence of self-critical, nihilistic and guilty thoughts, suicidal ideation, suspiciousness or paranoia, and perceptual abnormalities such as illusions or hallucinations. None of these symptoms are typically present or predominant in amnestic syndromes. Paranoid thinking is a common finding in individuals with dementia regardless of etiology. Marked depressive thought content and active suicideal ideation suggest pseudodementia but may also be present in early dementia where insight is intact.

Language. Disturbances of language are an important manifestation of brain disease, and the examiner should pay careful attention t each patient's spontaneous speech, noting errors and difficulties with fluency, grammar, vocabulary, and comprehension.

Construction. Disturbances of visual-spatial competence is an early and sensitive indicator of dementia. Test this skill by having the patient copy several designs such as a horizontal diamond, a two dimensional cube, and a three-dimensional pipe.

Praxis. The inability ot carry out purposeful movements on command, inhte absence of problems of comprejhension, muscular strength, or coordination is a motor apraxia and indicates brain dysfunction. The examiner can ask the patient to whistle or fold a piece of paper and place it on the desk. Apraxias are common in Alzheimer's disease and usually appear in the middle phase of the disease.

Abstraction. This is a higher cortical function that can be tested by similarities, differences, and proverbs. The patient's level of intelligence and education must be taken into consideration when findings are interpreted. The examiner should proceed from simple questions to more difficult ones. Examples of similarity and difference questions are: How are an apple and an orange alike? How are a tree and a fly a like? How are a midget and a child different? Generally speaking, patients with brain dysfunction will give concrete answers and may have difficulty switching from similarities to differences.

Calculations. The ability to calculate is considered to be a higher intellectual function which is compromised by brain disease such as dementia. Calculations can be tested by serial sevens and by simple addition (e.g. 4+5) and multiplication questions (e.g. 4*3). Interpretation of results must take educational level into consideration.

General Information. Questions should be asked in order of increased difficulty. Proceed by moving from the number of weeks in a year to more difficult inquiries about geography, politics, and literature may be constructed by the examiner and used with each patient. Interpretation will require judgement about the adequacy of responses in relationship to the patient's intelligence and level of education.

Insight. This can usually be tested by asking patients whether they think they have a problem, and if so, how they understand it. Insight will be severely impaired in delirium. Patients with dementia often state that they do not notice a problem with their memory even in the face of obvious impairment. It is not always clear whether this represents an pregenically or psychologically based form of denial.

An evaluation of psychosocial stresses should be under taken whenever there is an acute disturbance of mood, thinking, or behavior. This would include an inquiry into losses, recent trips or exposures to unfamiliar enviroments, changes in the location of the patient's living situation, changes in daily routine and changes in the patient's caretaking that may be causing excessive or deficient stimulation.

Table 3-2. ECT Anesthetics

AGENT	RESPONSE
Methohexital	Standard agent for ECT; rapid onset, brief duration; minimal postanesthesia confusion. Rapid recovery. Minimum required dose is lower in elderly patients.
Thiopental	Cardiovascular depression; longer duration of action than other meds
Etomidate	Myclonic jerks during the drug's onset of action; adrenal suppression; less cardiovascular depression; prefereable in patients with heart failure
Propofol	Pain on injection; antihypertensive and cardiac-rate-controlling properties may shorten seizures
Ketamine	Hypertension; tachycardia; psychotic symptoms (hallucination)

3.3 Pre-ECT Evaluation

Anesthesia Consultation is an important part of the pre-ECTevaluation, and cooperation between the ECT and anesthesia teams is essential (Swartz 1993) (Table3-2) Other consultations may be helpful (e.g. neurology, cardiology) if history, physical examination, or laboratory findings suggest that further evaluation is needed.

Patients are asked not to eat food or drink liquids after midnight the night before treatment because nausea occasionally occurs during anesthesia. Patients should shampoo their hair the night before and wash their face on treatment mornings.

On awakening in the morning, patients may brush their teeth and take the prescribed medicines with a sip of water. To avoid extra weakness or dizziness, insulin administration may be deferred until after the treatment.

A hospital patient changes into a loose gown; an outpatient comes to treatment wearing loose-fitting clothes. The patient is asked to empty the bladder and is then taken to the treatment room. Then have him or her lie down on the treatment bed. Whatever the physical locale, the ideal location for the practice ECT provides privacy, not only for the procedure itself but also for pre-and post-procedure evaluations.

The patient is connected to oximetry, cardiac, and blood pressure monitoring. The points of contact on the scalp for EEG and treatment electrodes are cleaned so as to reduce impedance. (Manly and Swartz 1994). A blood pressure cuff located below the knee is inflated above the systolic blood pressure. Through an intravenous line, the patient receives a short-acting anesthetic, and once asleep, the short-acting muscle relaxant succinylcholine permits visualization of the unmodified seizure in the isolated extremity.

A mouthguard is inserted, as succinylcholine does not prevent brisk contraction of the temporalis and masseter muscles with the stimulus.

3.4 Informed Consent

Physicians have informed patient for centuries about treatment options and have sought their written consent to procedures for more than a hundred years. Informed consent has changed in recent years form a formulation that emphasizes the disclosure of information into something closer to a risk assessment. The issue came to a head in 1966 in a New England Journal of Medicine article on informed consent written by Henry Beecher, a professor of anesthesiology at Harvard University.

In April 1974, State Representative John Vasconcellos introduced a bill, coded AB 4481, requiring that ECT could be given only after 1) the patient gives written informed consent; 2) the patient has the capacity to consent; 3) a relative has been given a thorough oral explanation; 4) all other treatments have been exhausted and the treatment is critically needed; 5) there has been a review by three appointed physicians who agree with the treating physician that the patient has the capacity to consent. Culver, Ferrell and Green (1980) were among the first to analyze the meaning and the limitations of informed consent procedures. They argued that a depressive mood disorder, even one with suicidal features, does not necessarily render patients incapable of making informed decisions about their care.

After briefing the patient about their care, an education videotape and their families to the procedures for ECT and to unambiguously document the information that has been presented to the patient when obtaining informed consent.

The following consent form unique to ECT should be used, as described by the APA (1990). At a minimum, this form should document the patient's understanding of the indications for ECT, the availability of alternative treatments, the risks of alternative benefits, and the expected duration of treatment and convalescence.

Figure 3-1: Consent for Electroconvulsive Therapy

Information: ECT, previously known as shock therapy, is a method for treating certain mental or emotional conditions by stimulating the brain electrically in order to produce a cerebral seizure. The procedure is carried out by doctors and nurses while the patient is fully asleep under general anesthesia.

Description of the Procedure: While the patient is laying on a stretcher, a needle is placed in a vein and an anesthetic medication is injected. After the patient is asleep, a muscle relaxing medication is then given through the same needle, and the patient si given pure oxygen through a mask. When the patient's muscle are relaxed, an electrical stimulus is briefly applied to the scalp in order to stimulate the brain into a period of intense, rhythmical, electrical activity. This seizure lasts 1 or 2 minutes and is accompanied by mild contractions of the muscles. When the seizure is over, the patient is taken to a recovery area and is observed by trained staff until he awakens usually in about 20 minutes. ECT is usually given every other day for about 6 to 12 treatments, although some patients may require more than 12 treatments to reach maximum improvement.

Risks of the Treatment: ECT is among the safest of medical treatments given under general anesthesia. The risk of death or serious injury with ECT is about 1 in 50,000 treatments.

The extremely rate deaths that do occur are usually due to cardiovascular complications.

Side Effects and Complications: Patients may be confused just after they awaken from ECT; this confusion generally clears up within an hour or so. Memory for recent events may be disturbed, and dates, names of friends, public events, addresses, and telephone numbers may be forgotten. In most patients, this memory difficulty goes away within a few days or weeks, although a very few may continue to experience memory problems for months or years afterwards. Certain treatment techniques prevent or minimize the occurrence of such memory problems (for example, brief-pulse, right unilateral ECT), and your doctor will discuss these options with you. No long-term effects of ECT on intellectual ability (IQ) or memory capacity have been found.

Results of Treatment: Although many patients experience significant improvement after a course of ECT, no specific treatment results can be promised. As is true with all medical treatments, some patients will recover quickly, some slowly, an a few might not recover at all. Even when recovery is complete, relapse is still possible. Medication therapy or maintenance ECT is often prescribed after a successful course of ECT in order to prevent such relapses.

Availability of Alternative Treatments: Medications and other therapies may be available to treat your particular condition, and it is possible that some of them might work as well as, or better than, ECT. The advantages and disadvantages of alternate therapies will be discussed with you by your doctor.

Right to Withdraw Consent: Even though a patient voluntarily signs an agreement to receive ECT, he may withdraw his consent at any times, even before the first treatment is given. Withdrawal of consent for ECT does not in any way prejudice the patient's continued treatment with the best alternative methods available.

Risks of Not Having Electroconvulsive Therapy as Recommended: It is possible that ECT may be more effective for your condition than any other available treatments, and that if you choose not to accept your doctor's recommendation to have ECT, you might experience a longer or more severe period of illness and disability. Medication and other therapies have their own risks and complications and may not be safer than ECT.

I, _____, have read the above description of the ECT treatment that has been recommended to me, and it has also been explained to me by ____, who has answered any questions any questions I had. I agree to have the treatments and understand that Dr. _____ will be in charge of administering the treatments.

Patient Signature _____ Date _____
Witness Signature _____ Date _____

3.5 Caffeine Pre-treatment

Another strategy for seizure prolongation is the intravenous administration of caffeine, 5 minutes before ECT (Coffey et al. 1987). That is why caffeine augmentation is not without risk. Cardiac-rate controlling agent may be required with caffeine, and the practitioner should exercise caution when using caffeine in patients with a history of cardiac ischemia or arrhythmia. The dose of caffeine ranges from 125 to 2,000 mg starting with lower doses and increasing at subsequent treatments as needed.

There is currently debate over whether caffeine lowers the seizure threshold or prolongs seizure duration or both (McCall et al.

1993) Rosenquist et al. (1994) examined the effects of caffeine pretreatment on several measure of seizure quality ad impact (postictal suppression, ictal EEG regularity, and heart rate response).

3.6 Pre-Treatment with Atropine

Although it has been routine practice for many years to attempt to attenuate or abolish the vagal effects of ECT by administering an anticholinergic agent such as atropine before treatment. A study of the effect of atropine premedication on the rate-pressure product recorded an unsurprisingly larger increase in this measure with atropine than with placebo, but the authors recommendation to avoid atropine for ECT premedication except prior to seizure threshold determination was not supported by evidence for any harmful effects of the increased rate-pressure product. The potentially fatal cardiac arrest that has been reported in patients receiving ECT without anticholinergic premedication would scarcely have been expected to occur. Atropine remains the drug of choice for attenuating or blocking the direct vagal effects on the heart during and immediately after the passage of the electrical stimulus and in the immediate postictal period: sinus bradycardia and arrest (and the consequent sharp drop in blood pressure), the atrial and junctional arrhythmias, and ventricular premature contractions during sinus bradycardia.

3.7 Medical Factors

Common medications that should be discontinued before ECT are listed in Table 3-3.

Table 3-3. Common medications that should be discontinued before ECT.

MEDICATIONS	INTERACTIONS with ECT
Reserpine	Severe hypotension
Echothiophate	Prolonged apnea
Theophylline	Prolonged seizures
Lithium	Increased risk of delirium
MAOI's	Possible cardiovascular Instability
Other antidepressants	Possible increase in cardiac risk and no evidence of additive effect
Benzodiazepines and anticonvulsants	Increased seizure threshold and possibly impaired efficacy

Also, antihypertensive regimens should be optimized before treatment to reduce the chance of a severe hypertensive reaction during treatment.

Most diabetic patients are more stable if the morning dose of insulin is held until after their treatment. The insulin requirements usually decreases as a diabetic patient recovers from depression, and blood glucose levels must be monitored frequently during the course of ECT.

Most psychotic drugs should be discontinued in preparation for ECT.

- Lithium may cause delirium when used con currently with ECT, and it should be withheld.
- Benzodiazepines are antagonistic to the ictal process and should be discontinued.
- Tricyclics make cardiovascular management more difficult and should be discontinued.
- Monoamine Oxidase Inhibitors (MAOI's) are typically withheld, although a 10-day washout period before ECT is unnecessary.
- In the patient with a pre-existing seizure disorder, anticonvulsant treatment should be maintained for patient safety and the elevated seizure threshold overridden with a higher intensity stimulus.

Patients with coronary artery disease may be pretreated with 1 inch of nitroglycerin paste applied to the chest or one sublingual squirt of nitroglycerin spray at least 30 minutes before ECT. Also, regularly prescribed cardiac medication (e.g. anti-hypertensives or digoxin) should be taken with a small sip of water 2 hours before ECT. Medications that should be avoided before ECT include diuretics (because of the increased risk of bladder rupture in patients with a full bladder).

3.8 Self–Assessment Questions

1) What measures of laboratory evaluation target the pre-ECT patient?

2) What measure should be taken in the care of a diabetic patient?

3) Describe how apraxias are common in Alzheimer's disease, especially in the middle phase of the disease.

4) When is a short-acting muscle relaxant delivered to the patient?

5) Who is responsible for introducing the practice of informed consent in a New England Journal of Medicine in 1966?

6) What measures brief the patient about their care before the ECT procedure?

7) Even though a patient voluntarily signs an agreement to receive ECT, when can he withdraw his consent?

8) What is the function of intravenous caffeine before ECT?

9) When is atropine used in ECT premedication?

10) In what manner should patients with coronary artery disease be pretreated at least 30 minutes before ECT?

Chapter Four

Treatment Procedure

4.1 ECT Equipment

The ECT equipment necessary for an ECT suite is well described in the report of the American Psychiatric Association (APA) Task Force on ECT (1990).

- Suction and oxygen are needed in both treatment and recovery areas.
- Pulse oximeters should be available for both treatment and recovery areas.
- An ECG oscilloscope and automatic blood pressure cuff should be located in the treatment room.
- A fully stocked drug and emergency equipment cabinet should be at hand in the treatment room, and responsible for deciding on which drugs to include should be shared by the psychiatric and anesthesia staff.
- A dental examination is necessary, especially for the elderly. Some dental conditions warrant the use of an individualized plastic bite, prepared by the dentist and

used in each treatment. It is similar to the mouth guard used by athletes in body-contact sports.

- The ECT device, with all necessary supplies (including a copy of the instruction manual for quick reference) should be located on a cart near the treatment stretcher.

No current treatment in psychiatry draws more public skepticism than electroconvulsive therapy (ECT).

Apply a blood pressure cuff and record baseline pressure. The same cuff will later be reinflated just before administration of succinylcholine to block this drug from the muscles distal to the cuff and permit safe observation of the unmodified seizure. If unilateral ECT is contemplated, the cuff should be applied initially to the arm ipsilateral to the placement of the unilateral treatment electrodes in order to document that a generalized, rather than a focal contralateral, seizure has occurred (Welch, 1982).

4.2 Electrode Placement

Apply treatment electrodes (see Figure 4-1). Self-stick ECG recording electrodes are applied precordially above and below the heart, with a third applied to the shoulder as a ground. The appropriate ECG leads are then connected and a baseline rhythm strip is obtained.

Disposable, pregelled, stick-on electrodes are applied for EEG monitoring.

The preparation of the scalp for stimulus delivery and electroencephalogram (EEG) monitoring is a crucial part of the ECT procedure. Frontal-to-mastoid electrodes on the same side of the head are often preferred for EEG monitoring during ECT because they produce a high-voltage, and can be placed contralateral to the treatment electrodes during unilateral ECT to verify that a generalized seizure has occurred. The same ground electrode applied for ECG monitoring can be used for the EEG.

Returning to the debates over electrode placement in ECT as a factor in reducing side effects, a series of trials began in the late 1950's that established a unilateral arrangement (both electrodes on the same side of the brain) as the position of choice (Sackeim 1987). Innovation in the area of electrode placement in order to spare non-motor parts of the brain. In this case the right side, supposedly to spare the dominant left hemisphere and at the same time to spare memory. Unilateral ECT is as effective as bilateral ECT in the treatment of depressions but produces a significant reduction in confusion and amnesia. It should be the treatment of choice for all outpatients and for those intellectual workers who must earn their living by retained knowledge.

Figure 4-1. Electrode Placement

Bilateral ECT should be considered for patients who are judged to be most seriously ill. For depressed patients, indicators of such severity include acute suicidality, poor nutritional status, and severe agitation or psychosis.

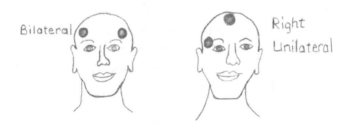

Douglas Goldman, who gave the first public demonstration of ECT in the United States at the 1940 annual meeting of the

American Psychiatric Association, also invented right unilateral ECT. His rationale for doing so was to avoid placement of the treatment electrodes over the speech areas of the dominant cerebral hemisphere (Abrams 1983). Thenon (1956) was the first to demonstrate the specific link between right unilateral electrode between right unilateral electrode placement and reduced memory loss and confusion.

This demonstration produced a ramp up the direct-current stimulus slowly until they got a convulsion on one side, then they increased the current-dose more until the fit spread to the opposite side. They noted that this technique was less effective than bilateral grand mal seizures. Some treatments advocate unilateral ECT at maximum energies and some bilateral ECT with dosing according to age.

Returning to the debate over electrode placement in ECT as a factor in reducing side effects, a series of trials began in the late 1950's that established a unilateral arrangement (both electrodes on the same side of the brain) as the position of choice. Innovation in the area of electrode placement in order to spare nonmotor parts of the brain (see Figure 4-1). In this case the right side, supposedly to spare the dominant left hemisphere and at the same time to spare memory.

Unilateral ECT is as effective as bilateral ECT in the treatment of depressions bit produces a significant reduction in confusion and amnesia. It should be the treatment of choice for all out patients and for those intellectual workers who must earn their living by retained knowledge.

Unilateral electrode placement should be used for patients very seriously depressed, but without potentially life-threatening complications of the illness. Unilateral ECT requires much higher doses than bi-temporal ECT to approach maximum efficacy.

Following placement of the stimulus electrodes and before delivery of the stimulus, adequate integrity of the electrical circuit should be documented by a self-test procedure. This procedure involves the passage of a small amount of current (below the patient's sensory threshold) to measure the impedance of the circuit.

Start an intravenous line. This step is most conveniently started with a 21-gauge, thin-walled butterfly needle assembly attached to a saline filled, 20mL syringe. Be sure not to start the intravenous line in the arm with the blood pressure cuff, because it will infiltrate when the cuff is inflated. Because I have deep, winding veins that make starting an intravenous line difficult to access, anesthesia residents attempt the procedure using an ultra sonic device. After multiple sticks if unsuccessful, the chief of anesthesia places the intravenous line in my neck vein.

Test Impedance. The static impedance reflects the quality fo the skin-to-electrode contact. An impedance of O suggests a short circuit between the 2 electrodes, sometimes formed by wet hair. A high impedance can be reduced by gently abrading the skin at the electrodes site.

4.3 Anesthetic Agents

There is significant variability in the dosing of anesthetic agents for ECT. (see Table 4-2 for a comparison of various agents used in ECT anesthesia). Administer atropine, 0.4 to 1.2 mg intravenously, by rapid bolus push. Patients with myocardial ischemia may benefit from a few minutes of oxygenation before anesthesia induction with the mask held slightly away from the nose and mouth to avoid a claustrophobic response.

Administer methohexital. This drug has become the standard anesthetic for ECT because it has rapid onset, has brief duration, and causes minimal post-anesthesia confusion. The minimum required dose is often lower in elderly patients. The answer to questions of how amnesia can be minimized is listed in Table 4-1. While the patient counts aloud from 1 to 100, and after determining that the needle is still patent and in the vein by gently aspirating the saline syringe and observing backflow of blood, replace the saline syringe with one containing an initial dose of methohexital, which is then given by rapid bolus push. As soon as the patient has stopped counting and is unresponsive to questions, the empty methohexital syringe is replaced by one containing an initial dose of 0.6 mg/kg succinylcholine.

The patient is asleep for 2 to 3 minutes and awakens gradually. Vital signs are monitored throughout the procedure. Systemic changes that may occur during ECT include:

- A brief episode of hypotension and bradycardia
- Followed by a sinus tachycardia
- Sympathetic hyperactivity
- And increase in blood pressure

These changes are transient and typically resolve over the course of minutes.

Table 4-1. how can amnesia be minimized?

- The change in electrical waveform from sine-wave to brief pulse square wave.
- Decreases in the total dose of the seizure-evoking stimulation
- Selective placement of electrodes
- Spacing of seizures
- Use of anesthetic agents to minimized the impact of seizures in memory
- Memory disturbances are usually not measurable for more than a short time after the end of a treatment series.

Table 4-2. ECT Anesthetics

AGENT	Usual Dose	Remarks
Methohexital	0.75-1.0	Standard agent for ECT; rapid recovery; pain on injection
Thiopental	2.0-5.0	Cardiovascular depression
Etomidate	0.2-0.3	Myoclonus; adrenal suppression; less cardiovascular depression
Propofol	2.0-3.0	Pain on injection; may shorten seizures
Ketamine	0.5-1.0	Hypertension; tachycardia; hallucinations

Methohexital has become the standard anesthetic for ECT because it has rapid onset, has brief duration, and causes minimal post anesthesia confusion. Another consideration is that the minimum required dose is often lower in elderly patients.

<u>Thiopental</u> has a longer duration of action and is more anticonvulsant than methohexital. This agent produced cardiac arrhythmias such as cardiovascular depression.

<u>Etomidate</u> is a good alternative anesthetic with low anticonvulsant properties. It has less negative effect on cardiac contractility than does methohexital and may be preferable in patients with heart failure. However, myoclonic jerks are often seen during the drug's onset of action.

<u>Propofol</u> has intrinsic antihypertensive and cardiac rate controlling properties, but the initial excitement over propofol as an ECT anesthetic has waned as a result of its excessive anticonvulsant properties.

<u>Ketamine</u> is interesting as an ECT anesthetic agent because of its proconvulsant properties. However, it is a compound related to phencyclidine (PCP) and can induce psychotic symptoms.

<u>Inflate the blood pressure cuff</u> to 10mm Hg above the systolic pressure to occlude the succinylcholine to be administered next from reaching the distal muscles (Fink and Johnson, 1982). This procedure is termed the "cuff technique" (Weiner et al, 1991).

<u>Muscular relaxation</u> is used during ECT to eliminate musculoskeletal injury and to aid in airway management. Administer succinylcholine by rapid bolus push. The empty syringe is then replaced with the saline syringe, and the tubing is flushed and clamped again for later availability in the event that additional intravenous therapy is required. Succinylcholine is typically given as a rapid intravenous bolus of a solution of 20mg/mL. However, a patent airway should be present before succinylcholine dosing, because the drug paralyzes the diaphragm.

Insert mouthguard and administer oxygen. The anesthetist should carefully evaluate the patient's mouth and airway before ECT for any potential problem areas. For example, loose teeth should be documented and may need extraction before the procedure. As soon as the succinylcholine has been given, a mouthguard is inserted between the teeth and 100% oxygen is administered by positive pressure and continued throughout the treatment (including the seizure) until spontaneous respirations have returned. It is prudent to oxygenate just before the procedure, especially in patients with a history of myocardial ischemia.

Observe muscular fasciculations of the first (depolarization) phase of succinylcholine. These will appear first in the muscles of the head, next, and upper chest and spread to those of the trunk and limbs before reaching the small muscles of the feet and hands. When the fasciculations have died down in the small muscles of the feet (generally about one minute after the succinylcholine injection), the patient is ready to be treated.

4.4 Treatment Stimulus

Administer the treatment stimulus. Seizure threshold is the minimum amount of electricity needed to induce a seizure. Because seizure threshold increases with age, the most commonly recommended system has been to select a dose based on the patient's age. When adequate muscle relaxation has been achieved and the stimulus set and treatment electrodes placed, oxygenation is temporarily interrupted, the patient's head and neck are hyperextended with the jaw held tightly shut a (properly inserted mouthguard prevents the tongue from protruding between the teeth) and the stimulus is administered. Like the electric paddles that cardiologists use to shock a fibrillating heart back into rhythm, ECT is not a mental health cure but can offer relief and even remission. Many patient prefer to think of ECT as somehow resetting the brain when it gets out of balance, the same way rebooting a balky computer sometime fixes it. Modern ECT devices use alternating current that delivers a stimulus in the form of a series of bidirectional square-wave pulses. This is referred to as a brief-pulse stimulus, which replaced the older ECT devices that delivered a sine-wave stimulus. The brief-pulse stimulus is more efficient at inducing seizures and consequently can produce seizures with a lower dose of electricity. This results in less cognitive impairment. The risk of injury to the patient of the practitioner from being shocked is very small. Theoretically, if the patient's impedance is too high, a skin burn at the electrode site can occur. This possibility is virtually eliminated by the provision of electrical self-test features in modern ECT devices, which allow the psychiatrist to check impedance before delivering the stimulus. The person delivering the stimulus is at no risk for getting shocked unless he or she actually touches the metal or the conducting surface of one of the stimulus electrodes. Calls of "stand clear!" are unnecessary. However, it is prudent to ensure that anesthesia personnel or other personnel do not touch the electrodes during the delivery of the stimulus.

In this chapter we review the recent studies into the relationship of electrical stimulus dosage and seizure threshold to the efficacy and adverse effects of ECT. Stimulus waveform refers to the shape of the electrical stimulus that is produced by a given ECT device.

Basic distinctions include whether the stimulus is sunisoidal or pulse and whether current flow is unidirectional or bidirectional. Sinusoidal waveforms were the first to be used; they involve a continuous flow of electrons in alternating positive and negative defelctions.

ECT devices also differ with respect to the mode in which the waveform is delivered-they may depend on principles of constant current, voltage, or energy (as fixed by the machine or set by the user) in the production of the electrical stimulus. ECT devices differ in terms the type of electrical stimulus that is actually delivered to the patient, with perhaps the most important distinction being that of waveform (sinusoidal versus brief pulse).

Charge is the best unit of measurement to describe the stimulus described as frequency, pulse with, duration, and current. Some ECT devices are calibrated in terms of joules, with the assumption that a patient's impedance will e close to the standard value of 220 ohms. This, patient seizure threshold may be expressed in terms of either charge or joules.

Several factors determine the stimulus, including the patient's medical condition, the type and amount of anesthesia given, and the urgency of the psychiatric illness. Because seizure threshold increases with age, the most commonly recommended system has been to select a dose based on the patient's age.

Following the electrical stimulus, there is an initial brief parasympathetic/ vagal discharge that can be accompanied by a brief period (several seconds) of asystole and a drop in blood pressure increase substantially, resulting in an increase in rate pressure product, which roughly correlates to myocardial oxygen demand. Other significant physiological changes include increased cerebral blood flow and intracranial pressure and a transient increase in intragastric pressure and intraocular pressure.

4.5 Observe the Seizure

Some of the patient characteristics and treatment factors affect seizure threshold.

<u>Gender.</u> Sex is a strong predictor of seizure threshold. Brief pulse stimulation, male subjects had a much higher seizure threshold

than female subjects, requiring an electrical dose that was approximately 70% higher to elicit seizures.

Age. A moderate association between increasing age and higher seizure threshold has been documented. In comparison to electrode placement and gender, age is the least critical factor in determining the minimal electrical dose needs to elicit adequate seizures. (Watterson 1945).

Diagnosis. Very little is known about how diagnosis interacts with seizure threshold. There have been a few reports suggesting that manic patients may have lower seizure threshold than depressed patients.

Medications. The impact of medications that could affect seizure threshold by either increasing or decreasing it. For example, a medication may raise the minimal seizure threshold, but have no effect on the duration or propagation of elicited seizures. In contrast, a drug such as phenytoin may have little impact on the minimal threshold, but may have strong anticonvulsant effects in terms of seizure propagation.

The seizure threshold often becomes elevated during the course of ECT. There is empirical evidence that this increase in threshold varies with electrode placement and cumulative number of treatments. Both the absolute and proportional increases in seizure threshold were greater with bilateral ECT than with right unilateral ECT Because bilateral ECT has a substantially higher threshold than right unilateral ECT, the stimulus dose often needs to be increased when patients switch from unilateral to bilateral ECT, if the dose is to exceed the seizure threshold by a constant amount. A large individual variation in electrical dose has been demonstrated at the seizure threshold.

It has been postulated that the efficacy of ECT is not a function of stimulus intensity itself, but rather of the degree to which the absolute intensity exceeds the seizure threshold. Studies examined whether adverse effects of ECT are a function of the absolute electrical dose administered or of the dose relative to the seizure threshold. With regard to the relation of stimulus intensity to the seizure threshold, the recent report by the American Psychiatric Association task Force on Electroconvulsive Therapy (1990) recommends adjusting the electrical dosage to the needs of the individual patient.

<u>What is observed in monitoring the seizure?</u> The tonic and clonic muscle contractions observed in the cuffed limb or EMG recording support the occurrence of a cerebral seizure. The electrical energy is individualized according to the patient's age, gender, and the type, amount and duration of medications prescribed. We deliver more energy to older patients than to younger ones and more to men than to women. The seizure threshold is the level of energy needed to stimulate a seizure. As patients age, the seizure threshold rises in a roughly linear correlation. The vast majority of ECT seizures last between 25 and 70 seconds. Seizures are a fairly common occurrence, particularly late in the course of treatment of an elderly patient.

When the patient is ready for stimulus delivery, the oxygen mask should be removed while a protective rubber bite block is inserted into the mouth. The bite block should be inserted so as to push the tongue inferiorly and posteriorly into the mouth, behind the teeth. Then the bite block should be placed against the upper teeth. Then the bite block should be placed against the upper teeth, and the lower teeth and jaw should be held up to firmly meet the bottom surface of the bite block. The chin should be pushed upward with firm pressure during the stimulus. After stimulus delivery, the bite block is removed.

The vast majority of ECT seizures last between 25 and 70 seconds. Seizures lasting less than 20 seconds are a fairly common occurrence, particularly late in the course of treatment of an elderly patient. Perhaps the most important reason to monitor the EEG during ECT is to assure that the seizure ends completely, because paroxysmal brain electrical activity commonly continues after motor activity has ended.

Prolonged seizures are now avoided by precise energy dosing and attention to anesthesia related to the patient's age. In fact, the electrical energy is individualized according to the patient's age, gender, and the type, amount and duration of medications prescribed. We deliver more energy to older patients than to younger ones and more to men than to women. The seizure threshold is the level of energy needed to stimulate a seizure. As patients age, the seizure threshold rises in a roughly linear correlation.

4.6 Self-Assessment Questions

1. What systemic changes may occur during ECT that are vital signs monitored throughout the procedure?

2. What is the most important reason to monitor the EEG during ECT?

3. What is the difference between electrical stimuli delivered during ECT of sine wave versus brief pulse?

4. What medication is given to block this drug from the muscles distal to the cuff and permit safe observation of the unmodified seizure?

5. Where are the ECG recording electrodes applied precordially?

6. How does the variation of applied treatment electrodes limit memory loss from ECT?

7. Why is methohexital chosen as the standard anesthetic for ECT?

8. What muscular fasciculations can be observed during the first (depolarization) phase of succinylcholine?

9. What measurement defines the minimum amount of electricity needed to induce a seizure during ECT?

10. What measurement takes place by the rise in the serum level of the peptide released into the blood with a seizure?

Chapter Five

Postictal Care

Patients must be carefully supervised and monitored by nursing staff during the immediate post-ECT period. Approximately 10% of patients will develop marked agitation and restlessness immediately postictally. This event usually is easily managed with a short-acting, rapid-onset benzodiazepine administered intravenously. Patients should be monitored for continuation of spontaneous respirations following administration of benzodiazepines in this setting.

After a seizure of any kind, whether artificially induced with an electrical stimulus or through pathology, the brain has a period of quiescence. That is, it becomes quiet, and its natural activity rests and recovers. All patients have some degree of confusion and disorientation immediately following ECT. This side effect is much more severe with bilateral ECT than with right unilateral ECT, and it may be more prolonged in elderly patients. Complaints of dizziness, shortness of breath, or chest pain should always be evaluated, and an electrocardiogram and cardiac enzymes should be obtained for any patient with significant changes in vital signs. During this time, it makes sense that we will not imprint memories well. It's also typical for patients to feel sleepy, not remember events surrounding the seizure, and even possibly suffer disorientation. This explains why the memory loss is most often temporary rather than long-term.

5.1 Seizure Length

After ECT, tardive seizures occur commonly in younger patients with a low seizure threshold. They are characterized by disorientation, agitation, combativeness, and absence. Seizures lasting less than 20 seconds are a fairly common occurrence, particularly late in the course of treatment of an elderly patient. A motor seizure of less than 20 seconds should prompt the following routine steps:

1. Decide whether to restimulate. Restimulation should ordinarily be attempted, unless there is some unusual overriding concern (e.g. development of a cardiovascular complication such as arrhythmia or severe hypertension).
2. Hyperventilate the patient vigorously for 60 seconds.
3. Reinsert the bite block, do a repeat impedance check, and re-stimulate at an approximately 50% higher stimulus level, or the maximum setting on the ECT device.
4. If the patient is to have additional treatments, thoroughly review the factors likely to have contributed to the short seizure (Table 5-1).

Table 5-1. Common factors contributing to the short seizure

1. Excessive anesthetic dose
2. A concurrent anticonvulsant, or another with anticonvulsant properties, such as a benzodiazepine or lidocaine
3. Lack of good hyperventilation
4. Inadequate electrical stimulus dose

Prolonged seizures are of greater concern than short seizures because of their potential to lead to adverse effects, particularly cognitive impairment.

Therefore, it is crucial to be vigilant for seizures lasting more than 2 or 3 minutes. The report of the APA Task Force on ECT (1990) states that seizures persisting for more than 180 seconds by motor and /or EEG criteria should be considered prolonged. Seizure prolongation should be determined by the EEG, because the most common occurrence is the continuation of EEG seizure activity after the motor seizure has ended (Table 5-2).

Table 5-2. Steps that should be taken in the case of a prolonged seizure.

1. Administer an anticonvulsant. We recommend giving approximately 50% of the dose of the anesthetic drug used. An alternative would be to give an intravenous benzodiazepine.
2. Continue to oxygenate (but not hyperventilate) and carefully monitor the cardiovascular status of the patient while watching the EEG for cessation of epileptiform activity.
3. If after 1-2 minutes the seizure is still ongoing, repeat the medication given above.
4. Continue pharmacological interventions along with full medical support of the patient until seizure activity is ended.

5.2 Cognitive Effect

The immediate cognitive effect after each seizure is confusion that is perceived immediately on awakening. However, within a very few minutes they are able to follow simple commands and then begin to speak. Table 5-3 summarizes reaction responses after the treatment. Speech is slurred, answers to questions are approximate, and orientation imperfect. The duration varies with age and physical status of the patient, with older patients in poor physical health having the greater impairments for longer periods. An example of how aging is important takes place as noted by Kitty Dukakis (2006) in a book she wrote about her experiences with ECT. Many patients in the text were referred for treatments were elderly and many most likely experienced regular "senior moments" of failed recall.

Initial disorientation and confusion generally subside within 10-20 minutes and typically are resolved within an hour. Approximately 10% of patients will develop marked agitation and restlessness immediately postictally. This event is easily managed with a short acting, rapid onset benzodiazepine.

5.3 Reaction After the Treatment

Table 5-3. Reaction after the treatment

- The patient usually breathes unassisted within three minutes after the treatment is completed.
- As he awakens, he is asked to give his name, date, and the name of the hospital.
- He may be puzzled by the questions at first, but awareness improves rapidly and his responses are usually correct within 15 minutes.
- After a half-hour, he is fully aware of his surroundings.
- Return to awareness may vary with the patient's age and the amount of sedating medicine he has taken.

- Within 15 minutes he is able to participate in normal daily activities.
- After the treatment, especially the older patient may be in a dreamy state, perhaps concerned about not knowing where he is or what is expected of him.

5.4 ECT Affect on Memory

After treatment, patients should always be rolled on their side to prevent aspiration of secretions and obstruction of the airway. There should be a staff member whose sole responsibility is to monitor the respirations and vital signs of recovering patients and prevent injury due to post-treatment agitation.

Occasionally, elderly patients become hypotensive immediately after treatment. This is particularly common in patients who are dehydrated from an extended depressive illness and who have not received adequate rehydration before their first treatment.

Numerous technical advances contribute to the modern art of ECT: the change in electrical waveform from sine-wave to brief-pulse square wave, decreases in the total dose of the seizure evoking stimulation, selective placement of electrodes, spacing of seizures, and use of anesthetic agents each has minimized the impact of seizures on memory.

The most known and feared side effect of ECT is impaired memory. ECT affects memory and cognition in three ways. It causes:

1. An acute postictal confusional state. All patients have some degree fo confusion and disorientation immediately following ECT. This side effect is much more severe

with bilateral ECT than with right unilateral ECT, and it may be more prolonged in elderly patients.

2. Anterograde memory dysfunction. This refers to the impaired ability to record new memories after receiving ECT.

3. Retrograde memory dysfunction. This refers to the forgetting of memories from the pre-ECT period.

5.5 Brain Location

Headache. A substantial proportion of patients report headache following ECT. This side effect may be related to the contraction of the temporalis and masseter muscles or to the cerebral hemodynamic changes that accompany the treatment. It is typically transient and responds well to acetaminophen, aspirin, or other nonsteroidal anti-inflammatory agents.

Muscle Aches. Diffuse myalgia's are most commonly seen after the first ECT session and then subside following subsequent treatments. These symptoms may be due to muscle fasciculation from succinylcholine.

Typically, the myalgia's are transient and respond well to the same symptomatic treatment used for headaches. If myalgia's persist after subsequent treatments and the patient's muscular block is adequate, the practitioner should consider lowering the succinylcholine dose or blocking fasciculation by pretreatment with low-dose curare.

Nausea. A minority of patients are nauseated after ECT. This side effect may be related to the anesthetic, the seizure itself, or air in the stomach from assisted ventilation.

When it is a regular occurrence, nausea may be treated with 6.25-25.0mg promethazine intramuscularly, before or immediately after ECT, before the patient awakens. Nausea may also be prevented by anticholinergic premedication.

Caution. The patient should be cautioned that major personal decisions should not be made during or immediately after a course of ECT. The patient probably should not drive until the cognitive effects of ECT have largely resolved and, in the case of continuation maintenance ECT, until 24 hours after treatment.

Finally, targeting the precise place in the brain where ECT is delivered demonstrates how the treatment works. Concentrating the seizure in the prefrontal cortex, the site of higher thinking is the best way to ensure that it is maximally effect. The left hemisphere of the brain is the primary center of verbal memory, so unilateral stimulation of the right hemisphere was introduced to minimize the direct effects of electrical stimulation to the brain centers of speech and memory. This is the best way to guard against cognitive damage, is to keep that seizure from spreading to other parts of the brain, especially to the temporal lobe, which is the center of smell, hearing, and short-term memory.

When it is regular occurrence, nausea may be treated with 6.25-25.0 mg promethazine intramuscularly, before or immediately after ECT, before the patients awakens. Nausea may also be prevented by anticholinergic premedication. Stabilization of vital signs within the margin of pre-ECT parameters in addition to return of alertness and orientation. After full recovery, patients are released to an accompanying adult. The patient and the post-ECT caretaker are advised that the patient should refrain from engaging in any activity that requires a high level of concentration or judgement, such as driving a car or operating machinery, for the rest of the day. The patient should be cautioned that major personal decisions should not be made during or immediately after a course of ECT.

5.6 Self-Assessment Questions

1. Describe care of patients who develop marked agitation and restlessness immediately postictally.

2. Describe the period of quiescence in the brain after a seizure of any kind.

3. What common factors contribute to the short seizure of less than 20 seconds?

4. What steps should be taken in the case of a prolonged seizure lasting more than 2 or 3 minutes?

5. Describe the three ways in which ECT affects memory and cognition.

6. How does concentrating the seizure in the prefrontal cortex demonstrate activities produced in the brain?

7. What muscles are involved in the production of the side effect of headache following ECT?

8. What premedication can be used to prevent nausea after ECT?

9. How long should a patient refrain from driving until the cognitive effects of ECT have resolved?

10. After treatment, what steps should be taken to monitor the patient in recovery?

Chapter Six

The Self-Vignette

6.1 The Clinical Problem

At 60 years old, I was admitted to the hospital with a severe melancholic depression of six months duration. In the hospital they gave me a very thorough physical to make sure my heart, lungs, and other organs could handle the procedure.

After talking to me during a visit, my son noticed that I was slightly drowsy. In addition, he found that the house was uncharacteristically dirty and there was a slight odor of urine in his mother's bedroom. My medical history was notable for hypertension and diabetes of many years duration, which have been controlled with medication. In addition, for the past 3 to 4 years, I also suffered from insomnia and anxiety, which have been difficult to treat.

At first I was treated with antidepressant medication. I tried Depakote, but gained 60-pounds during the first six months. When this proved ineffective, ECT was recommended. I consented and received an effective index course of treatment and my depression was relieved. I returned to an active life and was symptom-free for four years.

Then, without a clear precipitant, I again became depressed with severe sleep disturbance and attempted suicide. I was brought to the emergency department of the local hospital with cut wrists from a suicide attempt. The wounds were sutured, a blood transfusion given, and I was transferred to the psychiatric ward.

6.2 ECT Response

As an inpatient, I readily agreed to another course of ECT. It was significant that I expressed disappointment at failing to take my life, and stated that I was tired of living. Depression is a complex and heterogeneous disorder that comprises three broad domains of clinical manifestations: disorders of mood, cognitive function, and neuro-vegetative functions (i.e. energy, sleep, appetite, and sexual function).

I understand that ECT would almost certainly alleviate my depression as it had before, and I clearly preferred ECT to the options of no further treatment or combinations of anti-depressant medication and psycho-therapeutic support. After four treatments, my mood improved, my sleep pattern returned to normal, and my suicidal thoughts ceased. Both I and my family felt that I had returned to 80-90% of my baseline.

6.3 Maintenance ECT

In my personal experience with ECT, a needle was injected into my arm and I was told to count back form 100. Then a short-acting sleeping medication was injected sleeping medication was injected into the IV, and in less than thirty seconds later I was out cold.

A muscle relaxant was added to ensure that the only signal of my seizure will be a twitch of the toe. The anesthetic drugs left me unable to breathe on my own, so I was connected to a supply of pure oxygen that breathes for me and protects my brain.

Then the anesthesiologist inserted a plastic bite-block into my mouth to keep me from biting my tongue or cracking a tooth, a safeguard that works even better when a doctor or nurse grasps my chin just before the pulse is delivered. After the stimulus is applied, the seizure is indicated by a twitching of the toes or fingers.

The next thing I knew I was in the recovery room. I was slightly groggy and tired but not confused. However, my memory was slightly impaired. After my first round of ECT, the thoughts of suicide subsided and I went back on anti-depressants for a few more years. The return of symptoms led to a series of hospitalizations and medication trials to treat the depression I had been suffering from.

Later, I was subjected to an over-dose meds in a suicide attempt. At the hospital ER they pumped my stomach and treated me with charcoal. That treatment pulled me up enough out of the hole that I could function to go to my appointments, take my medication daily, and try to work with my doctors.

During the time of treatment the Depression and Bipolar Support Alliance calls it "an excellent option for people who have not found symptom cessation through any other method and who are deeply depressed and / or suicidal." Then I needed another index round, followed by ECT, maintenance therapy every 4 weeks. I'm not glad that I had the ECT but it's okay that I had it. I think if I got really depressed again and knew I was that depressed, I would give my permission to do it again.

Table 6-1. Methods of Suicide

Means of Injury	Percentage share for the year 1964
Sleeping Pills and other pharmaceuticals	12.4
Other solid and liquid poisons	3.3
Domestic Gas	0.4
Other Gases	10.8
Hanging and Strangulation	14.6
Drowning	2.6
Firearms and explosives	47.6
Cutting and Piercing instruments	1.9
Jumping from high places	3.7

6.4 Coping with ECT After-Effects

There's a predictability with this treatment that helps them to plan what my life will be like, and that makes getting ECT easier. That part I always remember a find reassuring. Just knowing what to expect helps me cope with ECT's after-effects.

- I know I sometimes get a slight headache, so I have Tylenol ready.
- I know I will be sleepy at first but will have enough energy to do things later in the day.
- Another way I used to compensate after ECT was not to drive the week after my first session. Once I get on

the road most things come back, from street names to turns I need to take.

- Memory loss: What embarrassed me most is forgetting people's names. My remembering someone may be only mildly important to them, but it is really important to me. Increasingly I feel comfortable admitting that I simply do not remember people's names. They assume its age related.

6.5 Follow-Up Care

Several medicine trials were unsuccessful in treating her bipolar disorder. The evaluation and treatment of this patient has been directed toward three goals:

1. A guarantee of patient safety involves evaluation and treating possible suicidal ideation (Figure 6-1).
2. A complete diagnostic evaluation to rule out medical, neurological, an pharmacological causes of depressive symptoms
3. A treatment plan should address not only the immediate symptoms but also the patient's prospective well-being.

First I was prescribed with carbamazepine (Tegretol), followed by valproate (Depakote), both of which were studied with rapid-cycling bipolar patients. Then I was treated with the selective serotonin reuptake inhibitor (SSRI) fluoxetine. That was associated with insomnia, nausea, anxiety, and headache.

I responded to Psychotherapy, which had its effects primarily on depressed mood, suicidal ideation, guilt, and social engagement. For that reason, combined drug therapy and psychotherapy was the treatment of choice. There were some concerns promoting ineffectiveness of all drug trials. Electroconvulsive therapy (ECT) was quite effective for both the acute manic and depressive phases of bipolar disorder. ECT was probably the treatment of choice, especially because was noncompliant with all medications and repeatedly suicidal.

My maintenance therapy was defined as treatments continuing beyond 6 months after the index course. I required maintenance ECT on a once-monthly basis. In addition, my treatments were shown to be very effective in preventing relapse.

Because many patients are treated with combined medication and ECT strategies during the maintenance phase, clozapine was introduced successfully to my care. Unfortunately, clozapine is associated with agranulocytosis, and because of this risk, I required weekly white blood cell testing. The period of highest risk was the first 6 months of treatment.

6.6 Suicidal Safety Plan

Step 1: Recognizing triggers and warning signs.

These signs indicate that I may be starting to get suicidal:

1. Hearing voices that tell me my life is not worth living and no one else can help
2. Involuntary movements of arms/ legs/ jaw become more pronounced
3. Crying a lot
4. Isolating
5. Stop showering and taking care of myself

Step 2: Using internal coping strategies

These activities may help me distract myself from thoughts about suicide:

1. Prayer/ Study the Bible
2. Talking to myself and using strategies learned in group to help manage the voice
3. Talking to family member
4. Exercising
5. Watching medical drama series on TV

Step 3: Social Contacts who may distract from the crisis.

These social activities and people may help me distract myself from thinking about suicide:

1. Mother and Father
2. Children
3. Group members at Psychotic Clinic

Step 4: Family or friends who may offer help.

These are people that I would be willing to talk to about my thoughts of suicide in order to help me stay safe:

Name and Phone Number

Step 5: Professional and agencies to contact for help

Therapist: Recovery Coach Primary care physician or psychiatrist

a) 24-hour emergency treatment
b) Call 911

  c)   Go to local Emergency Room
  d)   24-hour emergency Crisis Line

Step 6: Making the Environment safe.

These are steps I will take to limit access to means to kill myself:

1.   Have no guns at home
2.   I will take my medicine as prescribed and not over take them or under take them
3.   I will not drive
4.   Review the Safety Plan by keeping it available for easy access in a time of crisis.

6.7 Self-Assessment Questions

1. What affective disorder is associated with the highest likelihood of success with ECT?

2. What steps can be taken to make the home environment sage for a recovery patient?

3. Explain how age is the significant factor in the impact of ECT on memory.

4. What three broad domains of clinical manifestations characterize depression?

5. Explain how the placement of the electrodes affects the outcome of the treatment.

6. Explain how the release of brain hormones into the cerebrospinal fluid (CSF) and into the blood is the measure of brain seizure activity during ECT.

7. In a depressive mood disorder, what body functions are disrupted?

8. Why should benzodiazepines be tapered prior to ECT?

9. The minimal stimulus required to produce a seizure is the seizure threshold. What factors increase the seizure threshold?

10. What advances in anesthesia have been among the most important modifications to affect the safety and comfort of ECT?

Chapter Seven

ECT Discussion

7.1 Neurobiological Features

The pathophysiology of depression in late life appears to have some unique features. Susceptibility to depression in older adults is thought to be in part mediated by frontal-striatal-limbic dysfunction caused by vascular, neurochemical, neurodegenerative, and aging-related factors. The vascular depression hypothesis posits that vascular lesions in white matter disrupt key pathways, leading to a disconnected syndrome with abnormal functional activation in downstream cortical and limbic regions and resulting in impaired mood regulation, cognition, and neuro-vegetative function.

ECT for the treatment of psychiatric disorders is a form of therapy that has a range of effects on the neurobiological features of depression. ECT increases cortical GABA concentrations and enhances serotonergic function. It also affects the hypothalamic-pituitary-adrenal axis, normalizing the results of the dexamethasone suppression test.

ECT was first introduced as a treatment for psychiatric disorders in the 1930's. Early experience with the treatment raised concerns about serious side effects, including fractures (before the use of neuromuscular blocking agents) and cognitive impairment (in part related to dose and technique).

A guideline of the American Psychiatric Association Task Force on Electroconvulsive Therapy, which was published in 2001, includes a complete description of the current clinical use of ECT. In each case, a good response occurs with the need for a psychosis or a risk of suicide.

ECT is performed while the patient is under general anesthesia. Therefore, all patients must undergo a full evaluation by an anesthesiologist, including an assessment of the risk associated with anesthesia, before the start of ECT. Patients are not typically intubated, but mask ventilation with supplemental oxygen is used.

Neuro-muscular blocking agents are administered to prevent skeletal muscle contraction and possible injury during tonic-clonic activity. ECT was recommended for the patient described in the vignette for several reasons. ECT was appropriate given her lack of a response to or intolerance of adequate trials of antidepressant medications and neuroleptic agents. In addition, the presence of suicidal ideation with a plan for suicide underscores the need for a rapidly acting and definitive treatment. The presence of the psychotic subtype in the patient is a good prognostic indicator for a response to ECT, as is her age. It would be appropriate to consider starting with right unilateral ECT at an adequate dosage above the seizure threshold, but is she does not have a response, bilateral ECT could be used. Given the severity of her depression and her history of multiple episodes, it was recommended to combine ECT with an anti-depressant medication to prevent a relapse, tapering the ECT rather than abruptly discontinuing it on remission, and adding a mood stabilizer to the antidepressant to prevent a relapse. Maintenance ECT was also a reasonable strategy, and it was discussed with the patient and her family before the initiation of treatment.

The largest structure in the human brain is the cerebral cortex, the wrinkly walnut-shaped mass that sits atop and covers the rest of the brain. The cerebral cortex has four main areas, or lobes, on each side of the brain: frontal temporal, parietal, and occipital.

The frontal lobes consist of the motor cortex, which is in in charge of directing movement; the premotor cortex, which helps to plan movement; and the prefrontal cortex, which is the most evolved part of the human brain and is involved with focus, forethought, judgement, organization, planning, impulse control, empathy, and learning from mistakes.

The temporal lobes, located underneath your temples and behind your eyes, are involved in mood stability, emotional reactions, temper control, learning, moving memories into long-term storage, and auditory processing.

The parietal lobes, at the top side and back of the brain, are the centers for sensory processing (touch), perception, and sense of direction. They're also involved in manipulating numbers, dressing, and grooming. The occipital lobes, at the back of the cortex, are concerned primarily with vision and visual processing. Sitting underneath the cerebral cortex is the limbic or emotional system: the part of the brain that colors our emotions and is involved with bonding, nesting, feeding, sexuality, and emotions. Also underneath the cortex the basal ganglia, involved with motivation, pleasure, and smoothing motor movements. The cerebellum-at the back bottom part of the brain-is involved with motor and thought coordination. It is essential for processing complex information.

The cortex is divided into two hemispheres, left and right. While the two sides significantly overlap in function, the left side in right-handed people is generally the seat of language, and tends to be the analytical, logical, detail-oriented part of the brain, while the right hemisphere sees the big picture and is likely involved more with hunches and intuition. It is often opposite in left-handed people.

Many things help the brain. The exciting news is that many hinges are also good for your brain and can boost its function, such as learning new things; great nutrition; coordination exercises; meditation; loving relationships; and certain nutrients, including vitamins B6, B12, and D, and Omega-3 fatty acids.

When the brain's biology is healthy multiple factors work together to maximize success and sense of well-being. For example, when the patient does not get enough sleep, there is an overall decreased blood flow to the brain, which disrupts thinking, memory, and concentration. Likewise, a brain injury hurts the machinery of the brain, causing struggles with depression, thinking and memory issues, and temper problems.

7.2 Suicidal Patients

Use of firearms is the most common method of committing suicide for both men and women in the United States, accounting for nearly 60% of completed suicides. Hanging is the second most common method used by men, and drug in-gestation is the second most common method used by women. It is significant that drug ingestion accounts for approximately 70% of unsuccessful suicides. (Moscicki 1994).

Rates generally increase with age, because people over the age 65 are 1.5 times more likely to commit suicide than are younger individuals. Twenty percent of all suicides occur in the elderly, although they constitute only 13% of the population. One reason for this may be that the elderly appear to make more attempts that are more serious on their lives. It is documented that one of every four attempts in this group results in a completed suicide.

The examiner who interviews a patient after a suicide attempt needs to evaluate the details, seriousness, risk/rescue ratio, and precipitants of the attempt. The patient who carries out a detailed plan, who perceives the attempt as lethal, who thinks that death will be certain, who is disappointed to be alive, and who must face unchanged stressors will be at a continued high risk for suicide. The patient who makes a calculated, premeditated attempt may also be at a higher risk for a repeat attempt than the patient who makes a hasty, impulsive attempt (out of anger, a desire for revenge, or a desire for attention) or is intoxicated. (Hawton 1987, Fawcett et al 1993).

Certain populations of patients are substantially more likely to be considered for ECT than others, for good reason. People thinking about killing themselves top the list. The logic for using ECT as a first-choice treatment with suicidal patients is compelling. They need something faster acting than anti-depressants, which can take weeks to kick in. ECT generally starts working within a couple of treatments, meaning a couple of days.

Some reports showed that ECT does not prevent suicide. Others argued that it reduces overall mortality and suicide in particular. The newest and most exhaustive report on ECT and suicide offers convincing evidence that the therapy does produce a rapid if fleeting reduction in suicidal thinking.

If suicidality is the most compelling reason people turn to ECT, old age is a close second. One national survey showed that more than a third of hospitalized ECT patients are over sixty-five. Why the yawning age gap? It is partly that senior citizens suffer more major depression than other age groups, especially if they live in a nursing home, and suicide is much more common among older Americans.

It is tempting to attribute that to the facts that the elderly are well insured, physically and sometimes mentally frail, and therefore ripe for exploration. The truth is that older Americans suffer at higher rates precisely the forms of depression. Where ECT is most likely to be prescribed. They often have heart and other medical conditions that prevent their taking anti-depressants. This makes the elderly more likely to consider ECT. For the elderly, ECT's very success in treating depression can uncloak hidden dementia. Major depression is also the commonest cause of reversible dementia, and successful ECT treatment can lift the dementia along with the depression.

More than two out of three ECT patients are women. The gender difference is not surprising, since nearly twice as many women as men are diagnosed with depression, and depression is the most common condition for which ECT is prescribed.

More than two out of three ECT patients are women. The gender difference is not surprising, since nearly twice as many women as men are diagnosed with depression, and depression is the most common condition for which ECT is prescribed.

7.3 When does ECT Work?

The National Alliance on Mental Illness does not back any particular treatments but does acknowledge that ECT works, and says that nothing that works should be banned.

The American Psychiatric Association pointed in that direction when, in 2001, it urged that ECT be considered as the first rather than last treatment options for patients who are suicidal or suffer severe medical illness. Those results are convincing enough that doctors should think about turning to ECT earlier with their most deeply depressed patients. Table 7-1 lists indications for electroconvulsive therapy and Table 7-2 lists trials that failed and even had adverse consequences.

The indications for electroconvulsive therapy is used almost exclusively for the treatment of mood disorders and is generally reserved for patients who fail one or more trials of antidepressant medication, patients who are at high risk for suicide, and patients who are debilitated by their failure to take in adequate food and fluids.

Patients at high risk for suicide and in need of rapid treatment are also candidates for ECT because it tends to work more quickly than antidepressant medication. Research shows that approximately 70%-80% of depressed patients receiving ECT improve. Certain depressive symptoms are associated with a good response to ECT, including psychomotor agitation or retardation; nihilistic, somatic, or paranoid delusions; and acute onset of illness.

ECT is relatively ineffective in patients with chronic depression or in patients with severe personality disorders (e.g. borderline personality disorder). Schizophrenic patients are sometimes treated with ECT, particularly when a superimposed major depression or catatonic syndrome is present. Patients with schizophrenia of relatively brief duration (i.e. less than 18 months) who have not adequately responded to antipsychotic medication may respond to ECT.

The symptoms that predict a good response to ECT are those of major depression: anorexia, weight loss, early morning awakening, impaired concentration, pessimistic mood, motor restlessness, increased speech latency, constipation, and somatic or self-deprecatory delusions. These are exactly the same symptoms that constitute the indication for antidepressant drugs. The definition of drug failure varies with the individual patient; young, healthy, non-suicidal patients can safely receive four or more different drug regimens before moving to ECT, whereas older depressed patients may be unable to tolerate more than one drug trial.

Psychotic illness is the second indication for ECT. Case reports suggest that ECT in combination with an antipsychotic may result in sustained improvement in up to 80% of drug-resistant chronic schizophrenics. Mania is also known to respond well to ECT.

TABLE 7-1. Indications for Electroconvulsive Therapy (ECT)

- Medication-refractory depression
- Suicidal depression
- Depression accompanied by refusal to eat or take-in fluids
- Depression during pregnancy
- History of positive response to ECT
- Catatonic syndromes
- Acute forms of schizophrenia
- Mania unresponsive to mediation
- Psychotic or melancholic depression unresponsive to medication

Table 7-2. Behaviors for which ECT is ineffective

- Severe character pathology
- Substance abuse and dependence (including alcoholism)
- Sexual identification disorders
- Psychoneuroses (hysterical disorder, Briquet's syndrome, hypo-chondriasis, panic or anxiety disorders, pain syndromes, obsessive-compulsive disorders)
- Chronicity of illness without flagrant psychopathology

7.4 ECT Complications

That ECT causes complications is beyond dispute, although their nature and rates have been shifting over the decades. In the beginning, 40 percent of patients reported serious side effects like fractured bones and cracked teeth, most of which disappeared with the introduction of anesthesia, muscle relaxants, and a continuous supply of oxygen. The rate of serious medical injuries today is about one in ten thousand. A side effect of ECT that is far more frequent, and more difficult to measure, is the loss of memory. Difficulty recalling new information (anterograde amnesia) is usually experienced during the ECT series, but it normally resolves within a month after the last treatment. The most common, persistent, and hotly debated effect, called retrograde amnesia, involves the loss of memories starting around the time ECT is given and extending back months or even years. While advanced age, pre-electroshock difficulties in thinking and remembering, and confusion after waking up from early ECT sessions may predispose people to problems post-treatment, there still was no reliable way to predict whether a particular individual will come out of ECT with a worse memory.

The heart is physiologically stressed during ECT (Welch and Drop 1989). Cardiac work increases abruptly at the onset of the seizure initially because of sympathetic outflow from the diencephalon, through the spinal sympathetic tract, to the heart. This outflow persists for the duration of the seizure and is augmented by a rise in circulating catecholamine levels that peak about 3 minutes after the onset of seizure activity.

After the seizure ends, parasympathetic tone remains strong, often causing transient bradycardia and hypotension, with a return to baseline function in 5 to 10 minutes. The most common cardiac conditions that may worsen under this autonomic stimulus are ischemic heart disease, hypertension, congestive heart failure, and cardiac arrhythmia. For patients with coronary artery disease or hypertension, short acting intravenous Beta-blockers effectively reduce stress on the heart during ECT. Decomposition of congestive heart failure is usually treatable with oxygen and elevation of the head. It is extremely rare, but sometimes it becomes necessary to treat with intravenous furosemide and morphine.

7.5 ECT Risk Factors

A more frequent and fundamental question facing ECT physicians is whether the information they give potential patients adequately reflects the procedure's risks. To their credit, ECT doctors were among the first in medicine to use consent forms and make other efforts to inform patients, offering a model that today is standard with any surgery and probably should be with any psychotropic drug.

If questions about brain damage and consent to treatment form the front line in the battle between ECT's boosters and detractors, both sides increasingly are resorting to rearguard actions that impugn the other's motives and underlines its conflicts of interest.

As the technical conduct of ECT has improved, factors that were formerly considered contraindications have become relative risk factors. The prevailing view is that the following conditions warrant careful workup and management.

The heart is physiologically stressed during ECT. Cardiac work increases abruptly at the onset of the seizure initially because of sympathetic outflow from the diencephalon, through the spinal sympathetic tract, to the heart. This outflow persists for the duration of the seizure and is augmented by a rise in circulating catecholamine levels that peak about 3 minutes after the onset of seizure activity. After the seizure ends, parasympathetic tone remains strong, often causing transient bradycardia and hypotension, with a return to baseline function in 5 to 10 minutes.

The most common cardiac conditions that may worsen under this autonomic stimulus are ischemic heart disease, hypertension, congestive heart failure, and cardiac arrhythmia. These conditions, if properly managed, have proved to be surprisingly tolerant to ECT.

The brain is also physiologically stressed during ECT. Cerebral oxygen consumption approximately doubles, and cerebral blood flow increases several fold. Increases intracranial pressure and the permeability of the blood-brain barrier also develop. These acute changes may increase the risk of ECT in patients with a variety of neurological conditions.

7.6 Self-Assessment Questions

1) What is the difference between the times it takes antidepressants versus ECT?

2) Explain how congestive heart failure decompensates during ECT.

3) What does the vascular depression hypothesis posit in an ECT patient?

4) How does ECT's success in treating depression uncloak hidden dementia in elderly patients?

5) Explain how the heart is physiologically stressed during ECT.

6) Which behaviors document why ECT is ineffective treatment?

7) What psychoneuroses demonstrates clinical symptoms that are ineffective for ECT?

8) What symptoms persistent in the side effect of retrograde amnesia after ECT?

9) What frequent and fundamental questions face ECT physicians because of the procedure's risks?

10) Describe how the front line in the battle between ECT's boosters and detractors.

Chapter Eight

Geriatric Psychiatry

8.1 The Elderly Patient

The term geriatric stems from the Greek geras (old age) and iatros (physician) and thus refers to treating or healing older people. The life expectancy in the United States has increased from 47 years in 1900 to 75.8 years in 1996. Geriatric Psychiatry is one of the fastest growing and most exciting areas of clinical practice and research in psychiatry. It is of significance that older people may have coexisting chronic medical diseases and disabilities, may take many medications, and may show cognitive impairments. Those who study or care for elders will be challenged to be aware of issues of cultural diversity. In 1980, 12% of U.S. elders were Black, Hispanic, or Asian. In 1995, it was 15%, and by 2050, they will constitute about one third of U.S. seniors.

TABLE 8-1: The Physiology of Aging

- The blood volume falls with age, and there is a slight decline in hemoglobin concentration, more evident in women than men.

- Alterations in the cardiovascular system include an increase in the amount of fibrous tissue in the skeleton of the heart and in the myocardium and valves.

- Respiratory function changes with age and is complicated by the high prevalence of cigarette smoking. Totaling volume does not alter, but vital capacity falls and residual volume increases with age.

- In renal function, the glomerular filtration rate falls by approximately 1 % per year over the age of 40, as do tubular reabsorptive and secretory capacities.

- In the gastrointestinal tract, gastric atrophy becomes increasingly common as age advances.

- Age-related changes in hepatic mass and cellular structure are probably unimportant, but reduction in the hepatic metabolism of some drugs is well documented.

- In the bony skeleton it is uncertain whether osteoarthritic changes in many joints is an effect of age, the response of joints to time-related wear and tear, or a disease process unrelated of age.

- In the endocrine system there are minor declines in circulating thyroid hormone levels, a reduction in the rate of secretion of insulin in response to raised blood sugar levels, and a decline in insulin sensitivity.

- Age changes in the nervous system are among the most important, because of their great significance in the psychology of aging, and in the production of disorders of movement.

Advancing age is associated with a higher prevalence of both acute and chronic disease and an increasing risk of becoming functionally dependent. Roughly, 5.3% of adults between the ages of 65 and 75 require assistance with basic activities of daily living (bathing, dressing, walking, use of the toilet, and transferring from bed to chair). Slightly fewer than 6% require assistance with instrumental activities of daily living (cooking, shopping, use of the telephone, household chores, and handling household financial matters). Functional dependence greatly increases the need for both acute and chronic health care and amplifies the risk of institutionalization. A number of excellent reviews address problems and issues in assessment of older adults in a detailed and comprehensive manner. There are also good reviews about the neuropsychological aspects of assessment in the elderly.

Included below is a brief discussion of three salient assessment domains: cognitive function, affective status, and personality. A decline in cognitive functioning occurs during the middle and late adult years. The ensuing decades indicates that there is a general pattern of change in cognitive function across the late adult years, with consistent declines in perceptual motor skills, concept formation, complex memory tasks, ability to deal with novel tasks that are complex, and tasks that require quick decisions.

A critical problem in the assessment process is to determine whether any observed change in functioning is due to normal aging or whether it reflects some type of change within the central nervous system above and beyond what might be expected in the normal aging process.

For example, visual changes include decreased accommodation, decreased acuity, and decreased depth perception. Changes in hearing include a decline in high frequency speech perception and auditory discrimination; increased reaction time; and increased prevalence of nerve deafness, dizziness, and tinnitus. Hearing impairment may lead to heightened suspiciousness, if not frank paranoid thinking, and visual or hearing impairment may lead to a restriction in activity, social isolation, and loss of self-esteem.

8.2 Common Psychiatric Disorders in Old Age

This chapter highlights significant shifts in mood. Examples are listed in Table 8-2, as spices that boost brain activity.

Table 8-2: Spices to boost brain activity.

- Tumeric, found in curry, contains a chemical, curcumin, that has been shown to decrease the plaques in the brain thought to be responsible for Alzheimer's disease.
- A meta-analysis of studies found saffron extract to be as effective as antidepressant medication in treating people with major depression.
- Scientific evidence shows that rosemary, thyme, and sage help boost memory.
- Cinnamon has been shown to help attention and blood sugar. It is high in anti-oxidants and is a natural aphrodisiac.
- Garlic and oregano boost blood flow to the brain.
- Ginger, cayenne, and black pepper compounds boost metabolism and have an aphrodisiac effect.

Psychiatric disorders in old age include depression, strokes, Parkinson's disease, Huntington's chorea, delirium, and dementia. Complicating these diagnoses in elderly persons are the multiple medical problems that can mimic depression. Each section in the literature reviews the epidemiology, presentation, diagnosis, and treatment of the major psychiatric disorders affecting the geriatric population.

8.3 Mood Disorders

The disorder of mood commonly encountered in later life is depression (Hendrie and Crossett, 1990). However, depression in the elderly is often atypical and the diagnosis difficult. It depends on the demonstration of its cardinal features, such as loss of energy and interest, and a gloomy and despondent outlook on life and the future, with disturbance of sleep and appetite, and complaints of constipation and loneliness (Wells et al. 1989).

Depression is associated with low levels of certain neurotransmitters, especially norepinephrine, dopamine, and serotonin. These deficits can cause increased activity in the limbic system, which in turn causes many of the problems associated with depression. Since the limbic system is intimately tied to moods, when it is overactive the ensuing problems with depression may snowball and affect all the other limbic system functions.

There is a powerful connection between food and mood. Inflammation promoting diets are associated with depression and dementia, while anti-inflammatory diets are associated with improved mood, memory, and energy. The brain uses 20 to 30 percent of the calories that the patient consumes. Exercise dedicated as much as determined by all the right thoughts, meditate, and take dietary supplements, but if the patient continues to eat highly processed foods laden with sugar, bad fats, and salt, and made from ingredients grown with pesticides, flavored with artificial sweeteners, colored with artificial dyes.

Eat Clean Protein. Protein helps balance blood sugar and provides the necessary building blocks for brain health. It's critically important because it helps maintain lean muscle mass, which is a real issue as the patient ages. Great sources of protein include eggs, fish (wild, not farmed), lamb, turkey or chicken, raw nuts, and high-protein vegetables such as broccoli and spinach.

Eat Smart Carbohydrates. Carbs are divided into two categories: simple (which includes white breads, cake, etc.) and complex (whole plant foods, like green or starchy vegetables, fruits like blueberries and apples, etc.) Simple carbs, which have a high glycemic index, cause blood sugar to spike, while complex carbs have a lower glycemic index, are digested more slowly, are generally accompanied by other nutrients, and are higher in fiber.

A severely depressed elderly patient may be thought to be suffering from the irreversible brain changes that mark an Alzheimer's syndrome when, in fact, the memory deficits are the consequences of a severely depressed mood or the retardation of catatonia.

ECT seems to be particularly successful in treating severe depression in elderly patients. Most health care takes a holistic approach, believing that bodies need to be balanced physically, mentally, and spiritually. They include acupuncture, massage, meditation, yoga, tai chi, breathing exercises, herbs, and other methods to relieve tension and bring the body into balance. For example, some people use certain herbs, vitamins, and minerals (riboflavin, magnesium, and thiamine) in treating depression as well as anxiety. In biofeedback, a person learns to control their bodily reactions such as muscle tension, heart rate, breathing, skin temperature to stressful or upsetting situations. Guided imagery, or visualization, which involves going into a deep state of relaxation, is often used to treat depression, addiction, and anxiety.

Specific questions listed in Table 8-3 outline feelings of geriatric depression. Core symptoms include sadness, anhedonia, and crying. Other common associated symptoms are fatigue, insomnia, anorexia, guilt, self-blame, hopelessness, and helplessness. Diurnal features are that it is usually worse in the morning. Confusion and anxiety typically appear or grow worse at sundown, when the body is tired and the light is dim. This phenomenon is so common among elderly patients that doctors have a term for it –sundowning. Treatment focuses on bringing in familiar objects and family photos, and leave on low lights at night. Lots of visits and physical contact will reduce confusion.

TABLE 8-3. Geriatric Depression Scale

1. Are you satisfied with your life? No
2. Have you dropped May of your activities and interests? Yes
3. Do you feel that your life is empty? Yes
4. Do you often get bored? Yes
5. Are in good spirits most of the time? No
6. Are you afraid that something bad is going to happen to you? Yes
7. Do you feel happy most of the time? No
8. Do you often feel helpless? Yes
9. Do you prefer to stay at home, rather than going out and doing new things? Yes
10. Do you feel that you have more problems with memory than most people? Yes
11. Do you think it is wonderful to be alive now? No
12. Do you feel pretty worthless the way you are now? Yes
13. Do you feel full of energy? No
14. Do you feel that your situation is hopeless? Yes
15. Do you think that most people are better off than you are? Yes

---

Score one point for each indicated answer. A score greater than 5 indicates probable depression. (Yesavage, 1988).

Mania occurs in old age usually with a history of bipolar disorders. Extreme agitation or manic-like behavior can be caused by organic factors, dementia, schizophrenia, depression, or situational anxiety.

Symptoms of manic states can be described according to three stages: hypomania, acute mania, and delirious mania. Symptoms of mood, cognition and perception, and activity and behavior are presented for each stage.

Stage I: Hypomania. At this stage, the disturbance is not sufficiently severe to cause marked impairment in social or occupational functioning or to require hospitalization. The mood of a hypomanic person is cheerful and expansive. However, there is an underlying irritability that surfaces rapidly when the person's wishes and desires go unfulfilled. The nature of the hypomanic person is very volatile and fluctuating.

Perceptions of the "self" are exalted with ideas of great worth and ability. Thinking is flighty, with a rapid flow of ideas. Perception of the environment is heightened, but the individual is so easily distracted by irrelevant stimuli that goal-directed activities are difficult.

Hypomanic individuals exhibit increased motor activity. They are perceived as being very extroverted and sociable, and because of this they attract numerous acquaintances. However, they lack the depth of personality and warmth to formulate close friendships. They talk and laugh a lot, usually very loudly and often inappropriately. Increased libido is common. Some individuals experience anorexia and weight loss. The exalted self-perception leads some hypomanic to engage in inappropriate behaviors, such as phoning the President of the United States, or buying huge amounts on a credit card without having the resources to pay.

Stage II: Acute Mania. Symptoms of acute mania may be a progression in intensification of those experienced in hypomania, or they may be manifested directly. Most individuals experience marked impairment in functioning and require hospitalization. Acute mania is characterized by euphoria and elation. The person appears to be an a continuous high. However, the mood is always subject to frequent variation, easily changing to irritability and anger or even to sadness and crying. Cognition and perception become fragmented and often psychotic in acute mania. Rapid thinking proceeds to racing and disjointed thinking (flight of ideas) and may be manifested by a continuous flow of accelerated, pressured speech (loquaciousness), with abrupt changes from topic to topic. When flight of ideas is severe, speech may be disorganized and incoherent. Distractibility becomes all-pervasive. Attention can be diverted by even the smallest of stimuli. Hallucinations and delusions (usually paranoid and grandiose) are common.

Psychomotor activity is excessive. Sexual interest is increased. There is poor impulse control, and the individual who is normally discreet may become socially and sexuality uninhibited. Excessive spending is common. Individuals with acute mania have the ability to manipulate others to carry out their wishes, and if things go wrong, they can skillfully project responsibility for the failure onto others. Energy seems inexhaustible, and the need for sleep is diminished. They may go for many days without sleep and still not feel tired. Hygiene and grooming may be neglected. Dress may be disorganized, flamboyant, or bizarre, and the use of excessive make-up or jewelry is common.

Stage III: Delirious Mania. This condition is a grave form of the disorder characterized by severe clouding of consciousness and an intensification of the symptoms associated with acute mania. Delirious mania has become relatively rare since the availability of antipsychotic medication. The mood of the delirious person is very labile. They may exhibit feelings of despair, quickly converting to unrestrained merriment and ecstasy or becoming irritable or totally indifferent to the environment. Panic anxiety may be evident. Cognition and perception are characterized by a clouding of consciousness, with accompanying confusion, disorientation, and sometimes stupor. Other common manifestations include religiosity, delusions of grandeur or persecution, and auditory or visual hallucinations. The individual is extremely distractible and incoherent.

Psychomotor activity is frenzied and characterized by agitated, purposeless movements. The safety of these individuals is at stake unless this activity is curtailed. Exhaustion, injury to self or others, and eventually death could occur without intervention.

8.4 Schizophrenia and Other Late-life Psychoses

Usually there is life-long history of schizophrenic illness but, rarely, the stresses of old age can precipitate a first episode in a predisposed individual (long-standing schizoid or borderline functioning). Occasionally there is associated intellectual deterioration. A historical review of psychotic disorders is presented at Table 8-4.

Table 8-4. Historical Review of Psychotic Disorders

Eugen Bleuler	4 Fundamental symptoms: ambivalence, disturbance of association, disturbance of affect, and a preference for fantasy over reality (autism)
Ivan Pavlov	Saw schizophrenia as a generalized inhibition or chronic hypnotic state arising from excessive stimulation of nervous system weakened by hereditary or acquired damage.
Sigmund Freud	Believed that the content of schizophrenic speech confirmed his theories of the unconscious motivation of human behavior and the stages of psychosexual development.
Carl Jung	Favored concepts of unconscious motivation in human behavior and used word association to explore networks of related memories, events, interactions, and feelings.
Adolf Meyer	Considered schizophrenia as a reaction to a traumatic life situation, a view basic to his psycho-biological approach to all mental illness.
Harry Stack Sullivan	Stressed deeply disturbed interpersonal relationships as the basis for schizophrenia, rather than the intrapsychic mechanisms emphasized by the followers of Freud.

Heinz Hartmann	Related schizophrenic psychopathology to severe conflicts over controlled aggression, which can interfere with the development of autonomous ego functions and thus disturbed perception and disrupt logical thought and human relationships.
William and Karl Menninger	Together worked in many areas of psychiatric research, treatment, and education from World War I to the 1970's and they regarded schizophrenia less as an illness than as a reaction to stress.
Margaret Mahler	Noted that schizophrenic children's inordinate attachment to their mothers stunted their psychosocial abilities; from this observation she developed the concept of separation-individuation.
Theodore Lidz	Suggested that the schizophrenic patient develops his own egocentric over inclusiveness in order to adapt to that of his parents.
Ugo Cerletti	First used electroshock in 1938 as a way of producing convulsions, to alleviate psychosis, first in schizophrenia and then in manic-depressive psychosis.

The pattern of development of schizophrenia can be viewed in four phases.

Phase I: The Schizoid Personality. Individuals in this phase are indifferent to social relationships and having a very limited range of emotional experience and expression. They do not enjoy close relationships and prefer to be loners. In addition, they appear cold and aloof. Not all individuals who demonstrate the characteristics of schizoid personality will progress to schizophrenia.

Phase II: The Prodromal Phase. Characteristics of this phase include social withdrawal; impairment in role functioning; behavior that is peculiar or eccentric; neglect of personal hygiene and grooming; blunted or inappropriate affect; disturbances in communication; bizarre ideas; unusual perceptual experiences; and lack of initiative, interests, or energy. The length of this phase is highly variable, and may last for many years before deteriorating to the schizophrenic state.

Phase III: Schizophrenia. In the active phase of the disorder, psychotic symptoms are prominent. Characteristic symptoms involve two (or more) of the following, each present for a significant portion of time during a 1-month period. Continuous signs of the disturbance persist for at least six months:

- Delusions
- Hallucinations
- Disorganized speech (frequent derailment or incoherence)
- Grossly disorganized or catatonic behavior
- Negative symptoms (affective flattening, alogia, or avolition)

Continuous signs of the disturbance persist for at least 6 months.

Phase IV. Residual Phase. Schizophrenia is characterized by periods of remission and exacerbation. A residual phase usually follows an active phase of the illness. Symptoms during the residual phase are similar to those of the prodromal phase are similar to those of the prodromal phase, with flat affect and impairment in role functioning being prominent. Residual impairment often increases between episodes of active psychosis.

Neurotransmitter changes associated with aging may predispose to psychosis in the elderly. More specifically in the elderly, decrements in various neurotransmitter systems have been convincingly demonstrated. There are, for example, decrements in dopaminergic functioning associated with age-related cell loss in the substantia nigra, with or without overt parkinsonian symptomatology.

There are also age-relate changes in noradrenergic functioning associated with physical evidence of cellular loss in the locus ceruleus. Similarly, age-related cholinergic neurotransmitter system changes occur associated with decrease choline acetyltransferase enzyme activity. Collectively, these and other CNS neurochemical changes result in a resetting of the CNS neurotransmitter balance, and in many cases, these changes may predispose to psychosis in the elderly.

The Dopamine Hypothesis is a theory that suggests that schizophrenia (or schizophrenia-like symptoms) may be caused by an excess of activity may be related to increased production or release of dopamine at nerve terminals, increased receptor, or a combination of these mechanisms.

Pharmacological support for this hypothesis exists. Amphetamines, which increase levels of dopamine, induce psychotomimetic symptoms. Neuroleptic agents lower brain levels of dopamine by blocking dopamine receptors, thus reducing the schizophrenic symptoms, including those induced by amphetamines.

8.5 Paranoia

Mild suspiciousness among the elderly is very common. Bizarre forms or near psychotic levels may occur with:

1. Early dementia-always check for intellectual loss
2. Delirium
3. Vision or hearing problems
4. Social Isolation
5. Drugs-e.g. steroids, antiparkinsonians, hypnotic withdrawal.

Paranoid Schizophrenia is characterized mainly by the presence of delusions of persecution or grandeur and auditory hallucinations related to a single theme. The individual is often tense, suspicious, and guarded, and may be argumentative, hostile, and aggressive. Less regression of mental faculties, emotional response, and behavior is seen than in the other subtypes of schizophrenia. Social impairment may be minimal, and there is some evidence that prognosis, particularly with regard to occupational functioning and capacity for independent living, is promising.

Paranoid personality was first described by Adolf Meyer in the early twentieth century. Early formulations of the disorder came from a psychoanalytic perspective, which emphasized the defense mechanisms of reaction formation and projection. Some researchers have hypothesized that paranoid personality disorder lies within the schizophrenic spectrum and is the product of a common genetic predisposition. A behavioral model has been suggested in which suspiciousness and mistrust are learned, leading to social withdrawal, testing of others, and ruminative suspiciousness. These patients are chronically suspicious, distrust others, and fulfill their suspicious prophecies by leading others to be overly cautious and deceptive.

8.6 Delusional Disorders

These symptoms often have an onset late in life (late paraphrenia). Patients have fixed paranoid delusions and occasionally auditory hallucinations but not the loose associations, grandiosity, major hallucinations, and autistic thought of paranoid schizophrenics. Treat with reality-oriented psychotherapy, behavior modification, maintenance antipsychotics, and ECT.

The elderly are frequently ill and may develop a preoccupation with exaggerated physical complaints and problems. This is particularly common among depressed and /or demented elderly. That is why the physical symptoms may or may not improve with resolution of the depression. Hypochondriasis may be defined as an unrealistic or inaccurate interpretation of physical symptoms or sensations, leading to preoccupation and fear of having a serious disease. The fear becomes disabling and persists despite appropriate reassurance that nor organic pathology can be detected may be present, but in the individual with hypochondriasis, the symptoms are excessive in relation to the degree of pathology. They are profoundly are occupied with their bodies and are totally aware of even the slightest change in feeling or sensation. The preoccupation may be with a specific organ or disease (e.g. cardiac disease), with bodily functions (e.g. peristalsis or heartbeat), or even with minor physical alterations (e.g. a small sore or an occasional cough). Individuals with hypochondriasis may become convinced that a rapid heart rate indicates that they have heart disease or that the small sore is skin cancer.

Individuals with hypochondriasis often have a long history of doctor shopping and are convinced that they are not receiving proper care. Anxiety and depression are common, and obsessive-compulsive traits frequently accompany the disorder. Social and occupational functioning may be impaired because of the disorder.

Adjustment disorders are common in old age and are due to the numerous stresses (loss, physical illness, retirement, etc.) encountered. Alcohol abuse is also a common response to stress in the elderly and is frequently unrecognized. Other symptoms include anxiety, depression, agitation, and physical complaints and most often occur in persons with past adjustment problems. Table 8-5 presents the clinical findings of Adjustment disorders. Grief is also common and may mimic a major depression but often has an obvious precipitant, is short-lived with therapy, and does not require anti-depressants. Supportive psychotherapy, attention to concrete problems, and brief use of minor tranquilizers or low dose antipsychotics helps.

Table 8-5. Clinical Findings of Adjustment Disorders.

SUBTYPE	SYMPTOMS
Depressed mood	Dysphoria, tearfulness, and hopelessness
Anxiety	Psychic anxiety, palpitations, jitteriness, or hyperventilation
Conduct Disturbance	Violated rights of others, age-appropriate societal norms and rules are disregarded (vandalism, reckless driving, or fighting)
Work Disturbance	Difficulty functioning at work
Withdrawal	Socially withdrawn behavior that is to typical for the person.

In making the diagnosis of adjustment disorder, the crucial question is: what is the patient having trouble adjusting to? Without a stressor to cause maladjustment, no adjustment disorder is present. As with the assessment of any mental disorder, the patient being evaluated for an adjustment disorder should undergo a thorough physical examination and mental status examination to rule out alternative diagnoses. The differential diagnosis reflects the broad range of symptoms seen in adjustment disorders such as major depression; anxiety disorders such as panic disorder or generalized anxiety disorder; and conduct disorders. Personality disorders should be considered because they are frequently associated with mood instability and behavior problems. Patients with personality disorders typically react to stressful situations in maladaptive ways, so an additional diagnosis of adjustment disorder usually is unnecessary, unless the new reaction differs from their usual maladaptive pattern. Psychotic disorders are often preceded by the development of social withdrawal, work or academic inhibition, or dysphoria and need to be differentiated from adjustment disorders. Other psychiatric disorders that are believed to occur in reaction to a stressor also must be considered, including brief psychotic disorder, in which a person develops psychotic symptoms in response to a stressor; and acute stress disorder or post-traumatic stress disorder, which develops after a traumatic event that involves actual or threatened death or serious injury.

8.7 Clinical Problems in Old Age

Sexuality and the sexual needs of elderly people are frequently misunderstood, condemned, stereotyped, ridiculed, repressed, and ignored. "Use it or lose it" is a cliché that may hold some measure of truth. Interest in sexual activity in later years correlates highly with the amount of sexual activity in younger adulthood. Note that this finding is correlational and does not imply that having greater sexual activity when younger causes an individual to be sexually interested later. Factors that affect the expression of sexuality include the availability of a partner and one's physical health. Frequency of sexual relationships declines after 60 years but many men and women in their eighties and nineties are sexually active. The frequency and nature of sexual relations change with advancing age because of changing physiology. Men take longer to achieve an erection, and the erection is not as firm as it is in youth. Intercourse is still pleasurable, although the ability to ejaculate decreases after age 60. Following menopause, women experience atrophy of the vaginal mucosa, as well as a slower onset of lubrication. These changes may lead to dyspareunia (painful intercourse), but the capacity to achieve orgasm is usually maintained.

Many physical conditions also produce low sexual desire. For example, the sexual response of diabetic women is, to some extent, related to their blood glucose levels. Repeated yeast infections in the vagina and difficulties in lubrication resulting from diminution in blood flow produced by disease in blood vessels worsen this inhibition.

The sexual history requires asking the right questions. It is helpful for general questions to take the following form:

- Are you generally satisfied with you sexual relationship?
- Is there anything about your sexual relationship you would like to see change?
- How frequent do you have intercourse? What is your desired frequency?
- How would you describe the usual initiator of sexual interaction?
- What is the frequency of masturbation or the duration of foreplay?

Table 8-6. Classification of Sexual Dysfunctions

Sexual Response Phase	Phase-Related Dysfunction
Appetitive. This phase is distinct form any identified soley through physiology and reflects the patient's motivations, drives, and personality. It is characterized by sexual fantasies and the desire to have sex.	1. Hypoactive sexual desire disorder 2. Sexual aversion disorder
Excitement. This phase consists of an objective sense of pleasure and accompanying physiologic changes; importantly, penile erection in the male and vaginal lubrication in the female.	3. Female Sexual arousal disorder 4. Male erectile disorder
Orgasm. This phase consists of a peaking of sensual pleasure with release of sexual tension, and rhythmic contraction of the perineal muscles and pelvic reproductive organs.	5. Inhibited female orgasm (an orgasmia) 6. Inhibited male orgasm (retarded ejaculation) 7. Premature ejaculation (male)
Resolution. This phase entails a sense of general relaxation and muscle relaxation. During it, men are refractory to orgasm for a period of time that increases with age, whereas women are capable of having multiple orgasms without a refractory period.	No Dysfunctions

During the treatment phase of premature ejaculation, the man should initially abstain from intercourse. When sexual intercourse is recommended, the woman should be on top. At first the man should relax and permit intravaginal containment of his penis without thrusting. The woman should control pace and rhythm. Most men find that they have more control over ejaculation when lying on their backs.

Partners can use specific behavioral techniques to cure the problems of sexual dysfunction. The stop-go technique can be done alone or with a partner. The man is told to stimulate his penis to erection and to masturbate until he senses he is about to ejaculate. Just before reaching this point, he should stop the self-stimulation and wait for several minutes to let the intense sensation subside. He then repeats the procedure, bringing himself almost to ejaculation and then stopping. The exercise should continue for at least 15 minutes and include an approach to orgasm four separate times. By acquiring knowledge of his point of ejaculation and internalizing the body's responses to stimulation, he learns to control his timing and increase the pleasure for himself and his partner.

The squeeze technique also involves being brought to the point of ejaculatory inevitability. At this point the man or his partner applies a firm squeeze to the penis with the thumb and first two fingers. The fingers are placed on either side of the coronal ridge between the glans and the shaft of the penis. The squeeze should be firm enough to cause partial or complete loss of erection and should last for 15 to 20 seconds. After 1 minute, the penis should be stimulated again and the procedure followed as in the stop-go technique.

Sleep disturbances. Modern research supports findings of important changes in our understanding of sleep. According to these studies, sleep is a complex biological function whose length and depth is extremely variable: individuals may vary in their baseline sleep need between 4 and 10 hours. It takes the average person 15-20 minutes to fall asleep. Over the next 45 minutes, one descends to stage 3 and 4) deepest, largest stimulus needed to arouse). Approximately 45 minutes after stage 4, one gets to the first rapid eye movement (REM) period (average REM latency is 90 minutes). As the night progresses, each REM period gets longer and stages 3 and 4 disappear. Further into the night, persons sleep more lightly and dream (REM). Table 8-7 outlines the relationship between sleep and aging.

One of the fastest ways to hurt the brain is to get less than seven or eight hours of sleep at night. Chronic insomnia triples the risk of death from all causes and is associated with cognitive decline. Getting less than six hours of sleep at night has been associated with lower overall blood flow to the brain, and hurts mood, focus, and memory for days after. Fascinating new research has shown that the brain actually cleans or washes itself only during sleep. The brain has a specialized fluid system that helps to rid it of toxins that build-up during the day, including beta-amyloid plaques thought to be involved in Alzheimer's disease. Without healthy sleep, this waste clearance system doesn't have enough time to operate, thus allowing toxins to build up over time. Which can cause cognitive and emotional problems. Think of sleep deprivation's effect on the brain as what home or office might look like if no one bothered to take out the trash for a month.

Make sleep a priority and strive to get seven to eight hours night. Audio hypnosis can help with sleep. To help promote good sleep: eliminate or limit caffeine and alcohol; exercise in the morning rather than at night; turn off all blue-light –emitting devices (cell phones, tablets, e-readers, etc.) at night, and leave anything that will disrupt sleep outside the bedroom; make sure the bedroom is cool and as dark as possible. While studies don't advocate sleeping pills, supplements like melatonin and magnesium can be helpful for better sleep.

Table 8-7. Sleep and Aging

Subjective reports of elderly

a) Time in bed increases
b) Number of nocturnal awakenings increases
c) Total sleep time at night increases
d) Time to fall asleep increases
e) Dissatisfaction with sleep quality
f) Tired and sleep y in the daytime
g) More frequent napping

Objective evidence of age-related changes in sleep cycle

a) Reduced total REM
b) Reduced stages 3 and 4
c) Frequent awakenings
d) Reduced duration of nocturnal sleep
e) Need for daytime naps
f) Propensity for phase advance

Sleep disorders that are more common in the elderly

a) Nocturnal myoclonus
b) Restless leg syndrome
c) REM sleep behavior disturbance
d) Sleep apnea
e) Sundowning

Sleep disorders related to another mental disorder. This category was created to acknowledge that sleep disorders are regularly associated with specific mental illnesses, including psychotic, mood, and anxiety disorders, substance abuse conditions and personality.

Psychotic disorders. Patients with schizophrenia often report difficulty falling asleep, problems staying asleep, problems staying asleep, and impaired sleep quality. Studies of sleep architecture show a shortening of REM latency (i.e. REM sleep occurring earlier in the night), and a decrease in non-REM sleep slow wave sleep. Schizophrenic persons are also predisposed to a reversal in the phase of circadian rhythm in that there is a tendency to stay awake at night and sleep during the day. In addition, sever insomnia can be a prodromal symptom of an acute psychotic episode.

Delirium may lead to agitation, combativeness, and wandering during early evening or night time hours. Clinically, sleep may be fragmented with frequent awakenings, initial insomnia, or early morning awakenings. The studies find that sleep fragmentation, lower sleep efficiency, decreased stage 3 and 4 sleep, and a decreased percentage of REM sleep occur.

Mood disorders. Depressed patients report difficulty falling asleep, staying asleep, early morning awakening with an inability to return to sleep, disturbing dreams, nonrestorative sleep, and daytime fatigue and sedation. Findings form studies include prolonged sleep latency, increased nocturnal awakenings, and early morning awakenings. There is also diminished slow wave sleep (stages 3 and 4); and changes in REM sleep, including shortened REM latency and increased density of eye movements during REM sleep.

Manic and hypomanic patients may go without sleep or have shorter sleep duration because of their reduced need for sleep. The findings of studies are similar to those observed in depressed persons.

Anxiety Disorders. Patients with this condition are frequently associated with delayed sleep onset or trouble remaining asleep. Features from studies include nonspecific changes in sleep latency, decreased sleep efficiency, increased amounts of stage 1 and 2 sleep, and decreased slow wave sleep.

Specific anxiety disorders such as post-traumatic stress disorder, is associated with insomnia and other sleep disturbances. Recurrent nightmares are a hallmark of the disorder. Another specific findings are those of panic disorder, which may be associated with sudden awakenings from sleep, marginally increased sleep latency, and decreased sleep efficiency.

Substance Abuse. Alcohol dependence may lead to insomnia or excessive sleepiness. The effects of alcohol differ depending on its use. Acute use induces sleepiness and reduces wakefulness for the first 3-4 hours of sleep, with subsequent increases in wakefulness and anxiety-related dreams in the latter half of the night. With chronic alcohol use, sleep becomes fragmented, with short periods of deep sleep interrupted by brief arousal periods. Some alcoholic persons report an inability to fall asleep without alcohol. On discontinuation, sleep is initially disrupted; insomnia and nightmares may occur. Consequently, sleep improves over time, but light sleep and increased vulnerability to other sleep-disrupting factors may persist even after 2 or more weeks of abstinence. Studies in abstinent persons show a short sleep duration, prolonged sleep latency, and greater awake time during the night. There is a shortened REM latency, increased REM density, and a greater percentage of REM sleep during the night.

Personality Disorder. Borderline personality disorder (BPD) is characterized by mood instability, unstable relationships, and deliberate self-harm. Sleep studies have shown REM changes in persons with BPD are likely associated with the accompanying mood disturbance.

8.8 Self-Assessment Questions

1) What changes occur with hearing impairment due to aging?

2) What multiple medical problems can mimic depression in the geriatric population?

3) How does the blood volume respond to the physiology of aging?

4) What are the 4 fundamental symptoms of psychotic disorders described by Eugen Bleuler?

5) What are the stages of the sexual response cycle?

6) What disorder results occur when the brain's cellular aggregate known as the substantia nigra lacks dopamine?

7) What sleep disorders are more common in the elderly?

8) Explain how the preoccupation of hypochondriasis defines symptoms of illness.

9) How does the frequency and nature of sexual relations change with advancing age because of changing physiology?

10) Compare the difference in the clinical findings of Adjustment disorders in the subtype of depressed mood versus anxiety.

Chapter Nine

Psychiatry Treatments in the Elderly

9.1 Drug Use in the Elderly

Elderly Americans take large numbers of drugs. Studies of drug disposition in the elderly demonstrate wide heterogeneity in several important physiologic functions. Although drug absorption is unimpaired in general, distribution within the body compartments within the body compartments may be different in older than in younger subjects. Muscle mass, bone mass, body water, and some serum proteins are lower and body fat higher in older subjects.

Hepatic drug clearance depends on hepatic blood flow, serum protein binding, and the intrinsic capacity of the hepatocyte mass. The first two of these factors may decrease with age, resulting in impaired drug metabolism in some patients. Glomerular filtration rate (GFR) can fall approximately 30% from the third decade to the eighth. The fall in GFR may not be accompanied by a rise in serum creatinine because muscle mass is falling concomitantly.

Psychopharmaceutical treatment of geriatric patients requires special care. Table 9-1 lists Geriatric Drug Metabolism. Because renal and hepatic function both slow as a part of the normal aging process, medications for the geriatric population must often be given in smaller doses than those used for the general adult population. Start low and go slow is an excellent rule of thumb for psychoactive drug treatment of elders. At any given plasma level of medication, older patients have more side effects than their younger persons.

The FDA requires that all oral hypoglycemic drugs raise the possibility of increased risk of cardiovascular mortality. Further study has not convincingly demonstrated reduction in the microvascular complications of diabetes mellitus as a result of the use of these agents. No study has shown reduction in risk of blindness, renal failure, amputations, or death as a result of treating elderly diabetic patients with oral agents.

Table 9-1. Geriatric Drug Metabolism

The psychiatrist who prescribes medications to the older patient must be familiar with many factors that may affect the drug's effectiveness:

- Psychological changes with aging affect the pharmacokinetics may occur in the absorption, plasma protein binding, distribution, biotransformation, and elimination of the drug from the body.
- A decrease in the hepatic synthesis of albumin leads to reduced protein binding of medications and increases in the availability of free drug for entry into the brain or for access to metabolism in the liver.
- Since most psychotropic drugs are highly lipid-soluble, the amount of these drugs that accumulate of these drugs that accumulate in the body tends to increase with age for any given dose and body weight.

- Reduced clearance of drugs by the kidney affects medication that are water-soluble such as lithium or tricyclic anti-depressants, which continue to have cardiotoxic effects even after they have been oxidized by the liver to water-soluble metabolites.
- Reduced noradrenergic function with aging may render the older patients more susceptible to orthostatic blood pressure effects from tricyclic anti-depressants and antipsychotics.
- Reduced cholinergic function in the bowel and urinary retention, both of which are more common in older than in younger patients.

9.2 Anti-psychotic Medications

The changes in neurotransmitter systems in the elderly appear to play a major role, both in the etiology and the treatment of psychosis. Not only were agitated patients calmed, but the new drug seemed to diminish their terrifying hallucinations and troubling hallucinations and troubling delusional thoughts.

This group of drugs represents the major treatment for some of the most disturbed patients seen by psychiatrists. The major therapeutic effects of these drugs are seen during their use in acute psychoses. Effects include reduction of the positive symptoms, e.g. hallucinations, delusions, uncooperativeness, and thought disorder. Positive symptoms of schizophrenia respond consistently to antipsychotic drugs. Negative, or deficit symptoms, e.g. affective flattening, apathy, anhedonia, and blocking, are less responsive to these drugs. Antipsychotic drugs ameliorate and reduce the signs and symptoms of schizophrenia. Consider low potency antipsychotic drugs if patient is hyperactive or agitated. Consider high potency antipsychotic drugs if patient is withdrawn or lethargic.

Despite their effectiveness in treating psychotic syndromes, antipsychotics have the potential to induce a variety of troublesome side effects. The elderly are very sensitive to extrapyramidal (parkinsonian) side effects. Elderly patients have been known to stop speaking, ambulating, and swallowing as a result of these side effects. Partly as a result of age-related autonomic changes, the elderly also are highly susceptible to orthostatic side effects of antipsychotics. Falling may be associated with extrapyramidal side effects, orthostatic side effects, and sedating effects of antipsychotics.

9.3 Anti-depressant Medications

There are five broad categories of antidepressant drugs: the standard tricyclic compounds, the heterocyclic compounds, the selective serotonergic agents, the selective dopamine reuptake blockers, and the MAOIs. Each of the antidepressants has a different potency in blocking reuptake of one of the major central neurotransmitters: norepinephrine, serotonin, and dopamine. Important considerations in choosing an antidepressant drug are its relative sedative effect, anticholinergic effect, effect in seizure threshold, effects in cardiac function, and toxicity in overdose. An untreated depressive episode lasts 6 to 12 months on average. Because of that, the withdrawal of antidepressant medication before three months almost always results in the return of symptoms.

Tricyclic Antidepressants (TCAs) are believed to work by blocking the reuptake of both norepinephrine and serotonin at the presynaptic nerve ending. TCAs commonly cause sedation, orthostatic hypotension, and anti-cholinergic side effects such as constipation, urinary hesitancy, dry mouth, and visual blurring. Elderly patients should have their blood pressure carefully monitored because drug-induced hypotension can lead to falls and resultant fractures.

Another group of antidepressants, collectively known as the selective serotonin reuptake inhibitors (SSRIs) was developed in the late 1980s and early 1990s. Treatment should begin with one of the SSRIs because these drugs are effective, well tolerated, generally safe in overdose, and they have replaced the TCAs as first-line therapy. The SSRIs share a similar side effect profile. Commonly reported side effects include mild nausea, loose bowel movements, anxiety or hyperstimulation (which leads to jitteriness, restlessness, muscle tension, and insomnia), headache, insomnia, sedation, and increased sweating. These side effects tend to diminish over time and are largely dose related.

At about the same time that TCAs were synthesized, the anti-depressant properties of the monoamine oxidase inhibitors (MAOIs) were discovered. They inhibit the enzyme responsible for the degradation of tyramine, serotonin, dopamine, and norepinephrine. Blocking this enzymatic process leads to an increase in CNS levels of these monoamines. MAOIs are safe for use in the elderly when given with the usual precautions (see Table 9-2). Clinicians must record normal blood pressure and follow this stastic during treatment because MAOIs can cause hypertensive crisis if tyramine restricted diet is not followed. MAOIs also often cause orthostatic hypotension (direct drug side effect unrelated to diet). Relatively devoid of other side effects, although some patients may have insomnia or become irritable.

Table 9-2. Some Dietary Restrictions with MAOIs

Foods to Avoid	Usually safe	Unlikely to Pose Problems when Used in Moderation
Aged Cheese	Cottage Cheese, cream cheese, farmer cheese	Yogurt, sour cream
Beer, red wine, sherry, liqueurs	Vodka, gin, dry white wines	Other alcoholic beverages
Fermented sausage, beef or chicken livers, smoked or pickled fish, caviar	All fresh meat and fish	
Canned or overripe figs, whole banana peel fiber	Banana pulp	Other fruit, if not overripe
Fava or broad bean	Shelled beans, peas	Avocado, New Zealand spinach
Yeast/ Protein extracts		Soy sauce, chocolate, caffeine-containing beverages

9.4 Anti-anxiety Medications

Anxiety disorders are defined by a pathologic state characterized by a feeling of dread accompanied by somatic signs indicative of a hyperactive autonomic nervous system. The most frequently used class of drugs in the treatment of anxiety disorders are the benzodiazepines. There is no evidence of tolerance or a need to increase the dosage of the drug when such patients are receiving concomitant individual psychotherapy. Some of the anxiety disorders, such as post-traumatic stress disorder, are treated primarily with psychotherapy; others, such as phobia, generalized anxiety, panic disorder, and obsessive-compulsive disorder, are treated with a combination of modalities. The benzodiazepines produce few systemic side effects but can be lethal when combined with alcohol or other CNS depressants. The side effects of benzodiazepines are listed in Table 9-3. They may accumulate over time and cause sedation, confusion, and problems with concentration that are slow to clear.

Table 9-3. Side Effects of Benzodiazepines

Side Effects	Consequences
Sedative	Daytime sleepiness, impaired concentration
Amnestic	Mild forgetfulness, anterograde memory impairment
Psychomotor	Accidents, falls
Behavioral	Depression, agitation
Decreased CO_2 response	Worsening of sleep apnea and other obstructive pulmonary disorders
Withdrawal Syndrome	Dependence

9.5. Treating Insomnia

Older persons commonly report difficulty in initiating and maintaining sleep. They are inclined to spend more hours in bed and to experience fragmented, interrupted, and often unrefreshing sleep.

Subjective complaints may represent developmental changes associated with aging of the brain mechanisms that regulate sleep's timing and duration. Nocturnal awakenings and stage 1 sleep (lighter sleep) increase with age, while sleep efficiency and slow-wave sleep (stage 3 and 4, or delta sleep), which are associated with the refreshing function of sleep, decrease markedly with age. Therefore, the changes that occur with age represent not a decrease in the need for sleep, but rather an inability to consolidate an adequate amount of sleep during the night.

Primary sleep disorders such as sleep-disordered breathing (sleep apnea) and periodic leg movements of sleep (nocturnal myoclonus) are more common as people age. Both of these conditions cause increased arousals at night and impaired concentration and functioning during the day. Many elderly persons with subjective complaints of drowsiness during the day may be suffering from one of these disorders even in the absence of other symptoms.

Insomnia may be due to a variety of medical and psychological conditions. Congestive heart failure with nocturnal dyspnea and chronic obstructive pulmonary disease may make it difficult for the elderly person to lie comfortably flat in bed. Pain from arthritis, cancer, or bruxism, and nocturia from heart disease or urinary tract disease, may interrupt sleep. Mood and anxiety disorders, pathological bereavement, dementia, delirium, and substance abuse or withdrawal are common psychiatric disorders associated with insomnia. Older persons also commonly use medications that interfere with sleep. These include drugs with stimulant properties, such as the SSRIs and over-the counter decongestants. The beta-blockers may sometimes induce vivid dreaming that can cause awakening at night.

Sleep hygiene measures have been developed for patients with chronic insomnia. These measures include the following:

- Waking up and going to bed at the same time every day, even on weekends
- Avoiding long periods of wakefulness in bed
- Not using the bed as a place to read, watch television, or work
- Leaving the bed and not returning until drowsy if sleep does not begin within a set period (such as 20-30 minutes)
- Avoiding napping
- Exercising at least three or four times a week (but not in the evening if this interferes with sleep
- Discontinuing or reducing the consumption of alcohol, beverages containing caffeine, cigarettes, and sedative-hypnotic drugs

9.6 Psychotherapies

One of the fastest growing practices in psychiatry is the use of pharmacological agents in combination with individual or group psychotherapy. The common techniques that all psychotherapists seem to use include 1) offering reassurance and support, 2) desensitizing the client to distress, 3) encouraging adaptive functioning, and 4) offering understanding and insight.

The term individual psychotherapy covers a broad range of psychotherapeutic techniques. Both behavior therapy and cognitive therapy usually are done individually. (i.e. a single therapist working with a single patient). The historical roots of individual psychodynamic psychotherapy derive from Freudian psychodynamic approaches. Psychodynamic psychotherapy is used to treat patients with a variety of problems, including personality disorders, sexual dysfunctions, somatoform disorders, anxiety disorders, and mild depression.

The group approach to psychotherapy has established itself as a major form of psychiatric treatment. Group therapy provides patients with a social environment or even surrogate peer group that will help them learn new and constructive ways to interact with others in a controlled and supportive environment.

A variety of factors in these sessions include instilling hope, developing socializing skills, using imitative behavior, experiencing catharsis, imparting information, behaving altruistically be attempting to help other members of the group, experiencing a corrective recapitulation of the primary family group developing a sense of group cohesiveness, diminishing feelings of isolation, and learning through feedback how one's behavior affects others. Patients are typically carefully screened before being admitted to a psychotherapy group to ensure that they will be able to participate effectively.

Psychotherapy can help relieve depression in the elderly. Psychotherapy is especially beneficial for those who have endured major life stresses (such as loss of friends and family, home relocations, and health problems) or who prefer not to take medicine and have mild to moderate symptoms. It is also helpful for people who cannot take drugs because of side effects, interactions with other medicines, or other medical illnesses. Psychotherapy in older adults can address a broad range of functional and social consequences of depression. Many doctors recommend the use of psychotherapy in combination with antidepressant medicines.

9.7 Self-Assessment Questions

1) What three questions are required to support the individual prior to ECT?

2) What are the common side effects of the TCAs? SSRIs? MAOIs?

3) What are the commonly used anxiolytics? Indications? Contra-indications?

4) What guidelines should be required for gastrointestinal medication prior to ECT?

5) What special care is required for psychopharmaceutical treatment?

6) Explain how ECT affects memory/cognition in three ways.

7) What are the common extrapyramidal side effects that occur with antipsychotic? Describe the syndromes and discuss their clinical management.

8) What conditions represent an absolute contraindication to ECT?

9) What factors increase the seizure threshold during ECT?

10) Which drugs or foods will interact with an MAOI to produce a delirium?

Chapter Ten

ECT in the Medically Ill Elderly

Electroconvulsive therapy is known for its inherent safety, combined with an understanding of its medical physiology and its successful application in patients believed to be too old or too physically ill to undergo the stress of induced convulsions (Alexopoulos 1989). In this chapter the brain, heart, lungs, and endocrine system bear the brunt of the physiologic impact of ECT. Currently there are increasing numbers of patients who are elderly, frail, and suffering from complex medical conditions. Table 10-1 lists these functions as they present at greatest risk during the procedure.

Table 10-1. ECT in the Medically Ill Elderly

Central Nervous System Diseases

- Dementing Disorders
- Delirium
- Amnestic Disorders
- Brain Tumors
- Stroke Syndromes
- Epilepsy

Cardiovascular Diseases

- Hypertension
- Myocardial Infarction
- Cardiac Arrhythmias
- Congestive Heart Failure

Pulmonary Diseases

- Asthma
- Pneumonia
- Chronic Obstructive Pulmonary Disease (COPD)

Endocrine Diseases

- Diabetes Mellitus
- Cushing's Syndrome
- Addison's Disease
- Thyroid Disorders

10.1 Central Nervous System Diseases

Dementing Disorders. Dementia is a global impairment of intellect without impaired consciousness. These patients have an enormous socioeconomic impact on the health care system because they require such great amounts of care. Also, as the population ages, the number of demented persons increases geometrically.

Normal aging is associated with a decreased ability to learn new material and a slowing of thought processes. In addition, there is a syndrome of benign senescent forgetfulness, which does not show a progressively deteriorating course. However, neither of these includes an impairment in social or occupational functioning, which is part of the definition of dementia.

At least one of the following findings must be present in the diagnostic features of dementia: aphasia (language disturbance), apraxia (impaired ability to perform motor activities despite intact motor function),agnosia (failure to recognize or identify objects despite intact sensory function), or disturbances of executive function (including the ability to think abstractly as well as to plan, initiate, sequence, monitor, and stop complex behavior). The cognitive deficits must be sufficiently severe to cause impairment in occupational or social functioning. The diagnosis of dementia should not be made unless it is clear that the cognitive status of the individual has declined from a previously higher level of function.

If a person has dementia, the family should be aware of other problems that can exacerbate the symptoms (or cause confusion on their own). For example, depression can mimic early Alzheimer's, or it can coincide with dementia, especially in the early stages. Frustrated and saddened by the symptoms of dementia, people often become depressed. However, depression will only worsen forgetfulness, confusion, and other symptoms. Identifying and treating depression—and it is extremely treatable—can noticeably alleviate early confusion and memory loss. Be on the lookout for delirium because when someone with dementia becomes sick with some other ailment, and especially if he is moved to a hospital, he is apt to become delirious. Symptoms vary widely but often include disorientation, inattentiveness, and changes in personality. That is why antidepressants, heart medications, anti-inflammatory drugs, sleeping pills, ulcer medication, insulin, and cold medications can all cause confusion, agitation, and other symptoms. These medications or age can impede a body's absorption of vitaminB-12, causing fatigue, depression, anxiety, memory loss, and other problems typical of dementia. The deficiency is treated with injections of the vitamin.

Depression is common at early stages of dementia and may frequently herald dementia onset. The emergence of depression at any stage during dementia is usually associated with worsening cognitive performance and deteriorating function. Even when depressed mood is not evident, anxiety, sleep disturbance, or psychosis may be responsive to antidepressants.

The prognosis is excellent with depressive dementia, and virtually all patients shoe improvement after ECT. It has become clear in recent years that depression complicates the course of dementing illness in a substantial percentage of patients. The differences between these conditions are summarized in Table 10-2.

Table 10-2. Differential Diagnosis of Dementia and Dementia of Depression

	DEMENTIA	**DEMENTIA of DEPRESSION**
Duration	Months, Years	Days, Weeks
Past History	Systemic Illness	Affective Illness
Neurological Features	Dysphasia, Dyspraxia, Incontinence	Usually Absent
Answers to Questions	Erroneous, Confabulated	Often. I Don't Know
CT, EEG	Often Abnormal	Usually Normal
Response to Antidepressant	Usually Modest	Positive

Alzheimer's Disease. The classic gross neuroanatomical observation of a brain from a patient with Alzheimer's Disease is diffuse atrophy with flattened cortical sulci and enlarged cerebral ventricles. Understanding the molecular basis of the amyloid deposits that are a hallmark of the disorder's neuropathology. The neurotransmitters that are most often implicated in this pathophysiological condition are acetylcholine and norepinephrine, both of which are hypothesized to be hypoactive in Alzheimer's disease.

Alzheimer's disease is the most common disease which causes dementia. Traditionally, patients with Alzheimer's disease have been subclassified into presenile and senile types, depending on whether they are under or over 65 years of age. This disease can begin around 40, but the peak incidence of onset appears to be between 65 and 70. The early clinical changes in Alzheimer's disease are insidious, and family members have trouble even in retrospect in dating onset. For example, problems with memory are typically cited by the family as the first noticeable abnormality. As the disease progresses, there are increasing difficulties with attention, language, orientation, visuospatial skills, abstract reasoning, personality, and emotions. The gait becomes abnormal even with parkinsonism characteristics. The patient ends up bedridden and typically dies of aspiration or infection.

Vascular Dementia. This is the second major cause of dementia in the elderly. It occurs most frequently in conjunction with Alzheimer's disease. However, it is believed to be the result of cerebral infarctions of varying size in multiple brain regions. Conditions associated with cerebral infarction, such as cardiac arrhythmias and hypertension, predispose to vascular dementia. Vascular dementia is most common in men, especially those with pre-existing hypertension or other cardiovascular risk factors.

The primary cause of vascular dementia, formerly referred to as multi-infarct dementia, is presumed to be multiple cerebral vascular disease, resulting in a symptom pattern of dementia.

The clinical presentation of vascular dementia is more diverse than that of Alzheimer's disease. The disorder affects primarily small and medium sized cerebral vessels, which undergo infarction and produce multiple parenchymal lesions spread over wide areas of the brain. Speech disturbance or gait disturbance, for example, may occur at varying points in the evolution of vascular dementia pathology, whereas in Alzheimer's disease these deficits tend to occur at a specific point in the evolution of the dementia process. Most significantly, psychiatric disturbances occurring in vascular dementia include general dementia related psychiatric conditions, such as the affective, psychotic, and agitation disturbances described at each stage of Alzheimer's disease. Emotional changes characteristic of stroke-related dementia also occur, e.g. emotional incontinence and other sudden, labile, mood changes.

Pick's Disease represents a rare disease which is commonly confused with Alzheimer's Disease. Changes in personality and behavioral control represent some of the earliest signs of the disorder. Language difficulties, rather than memory problems, are commonly the first reported cognitive changes. The language problems are typically anomias, paraphasic errors, and word-finding problems. As the disease progresses and more global cognitive deficits occur, memory functions may be more spared. Pathologic changes appear to occur mostly in the anterior frontal and temporal lobes. Neuropathology of this disorder was recently termed frontotemporal dementia.

Creutzfeldt-Jakob Disease. This rapidly progressive degenerative dementing disease is caused by a transmissible slow virus. The disease is distinguished from Alzheimer's disease by its course, which may be more rapid, or by the occurrence of focal and localized neural pathology. The latter includes cranial nerve signs, such as auditory deficits associated with 8th nerve involvement, and gait disturbance, associated with cerebellar involvement.

Huntington's Chorea. This disease, distinguished by the triad of dominant inheritance, choreoathetosis, and dementia, commemorates the name of George Huntington, a medial practitioner of Pomeroy, Ohio. In the biochemical defects in Huntington chorea, the impaired glucose metabolism is in the caudate nucleus. Since at least a partial explanation for L-dopa induced involuntary movements is an excess of dopamine (in contrast to Parkinson's Disease, in which there is a decrease).

Memory is affected early and may be a sensitive predictor of the illness in individuals who are genetically at risk. Psychological disturbances, especially depression and suicide, are common. Dementia is also a characteristic of Huntington's disease, which is an autosomal-dominant inheritable condition localized to chromosome 4. Huntington's disease, accounting for 3%of all dementias, is an autosomal dominant disorder with 100% penetrance in which there is progressive neurological deterioration characterized by involuntary choreiform movements and dementia.

While family history and physical examination usually reveal the diagnosis, personality change, emotional disturbances, and cognitive decline can precede the motor abnormalities which may begin as late as the sixth to eight decade. Such a late-onset course can make diagnosis in the elderly difficult, especially when the family history may be obscured by ancestors who have died of other causes before the clinical expression of the disease is apparent.

Normal Pressure hydrocephalus. This condition is marked by gait disturbance, urinary incontinence, and dilated cerebral ventricles out of proportion to the magnitude of cortical atrophy and dementia. Urinary incontinence, neuroradiologic findings, and the relatively early appearance of gait disturbance assist in distinguishing this condition clinically from Alzheimer's disease.

Parkinson's disease. James Parkinson first cogently described this common disease, known since ancient times, in 1817. In his words, it is characterized by involuntary tremulous motion, with lessened muscular power. His essay contains no reference to rigidity or to slowness of movement, because it stresses unduly the reduction in muscular power.

The marked degeneration of dopaminergic neurons of the nigrostriatal pathway, and the severe reduction of striatal dopamine replacement therapy in Parkinson's disease. The most frequently employed treatment involves administration of levodopa, a precursor of dopamine able to cross the blood-brain barrier. It reduces the severity of the motor disorder and improves perceived quality of life in the majority of treated patients, although it does not appear to modify the progression of disease or change prognosis. The fact that ECT has clear anti-parkinsonian effects argues strongly for dopaminergic enhancement.

Parkinsonism is a clinical symptom presenting the following features: resting tremor (rhythmically alternating contractions of a given muscle group), rigidity (increased resistance to passive joint movement), akinesia (disability or slowness in initiating movements, masked facies, decreased associated movements, e.g. arm-swinging while walking and stooped posture), and loss of normal postural reflexes. A growing literature supports the use of ECT for the treatment of both depression and the Parkinson's disease (Andersen et al. 1987) (see Table 10-3).

Parkinsonism is marked by a progressive course described in terms of sequential stages. Stage 1 typically involves unilateral motor signs with akinesia and rigidity; Stage 2 manifests with bilateral motor signs and includes tremor and some alteration of postural reflexes; in Stage 3, a marked loss of postural reflexes occurs; and in Stage 4, the parkinsonian patient is typically able to walk only with the assistance of a walker. As the disorder of movement worsens, the voice softens and the speech seems hurried and monotonous until the patient only whispers. The consumption of a meal takes an hour because each morsel of food must be swallowed before the next bite is taken.

Table 10-3. Depression and Parkinson's disease

- Depression is present in about 40% of Parkinson's patients.
- Depression in Parkinson's disease is characterized by high anxiety and low self-punitive ideation compared with other depressive disorders.
- Risk factors for depression in Parkinson's disease are low CSF 5-HIAA and past depression history.
- Depression in Parkinson's disease is associated with bradykinesia and gait impairment more than tremor.
- Depressed Parkinson's disease have greater frontal lobe dysfunction than do non-depressed Parkinson's patients.
- Depressed Parkinson's disease patients respond to tricyclics, bupropion, or ECT.

Delirium is an organic brain syndrome of acute or subacute onset in which immediate recall as well as both short and long-term memory are impaired and accompanied by a disturbance of consciousness. The causes of delirium encompass the spectrum of most medical conditions including postoperative states, drug intoxication, and drug withdrawal. A careful review of medications should be undertaken since drug effects and toxicity, particularly anticholinergic toxicity, are frequent causes of delirium in the elderly. Important predisposing factors are advanced age, organ brain disease, and addiction to alcohol or drugs.

Delirious patients may appear drowsy or hyperalert (hypervigilant), trail off in the middle of sentences, fail to answer questions or ask that questions be repeated, or appear perplexed. Elderly patients who show no signs of confusion at home may become disoriented, argumentative, and forgetful in the hospital, and those who already suffer from dementia often become more muddled. Treatment begins with familiar objects and family photos, and leaving on low lights at night. Lots of visits and physical contact will reassure the patient and reduce confusion. If he becomes confused or agitated, the family members should remain calm because their mood will affect his.

Conditions most commonly present with altered mental state in the elderly are delirium and dementia. (Lipowski 1989). In delirium, there is impaired sensorium (reduced level of consciousness). Delirium usually has rapid onset, brief duration, and marked fluctuation throughout the day. The clinical course is characteristically a fluctuating one changing from hour to hour, or day to day.

Diurnal features are that it usually is worse in the evening and night, a phenomenon known as sundowning. Thus, it is possible for patients with delirium to have long periods during which their level of consciousness is intact and when other associated symptoms are absent. (Bross 1994).

In attention, distractibility, disorientation, and marked disruption of the sleep-wake cycle occur. The latter is often characterized by wakefulness at night and drowsiness during the day. However, even daytime somnolence is usually interrupted by periods of restlessness and agitation (Tueth 1993).

Mood lability, incoherent speech, disorganized thinking, and perceptual disturbances, such as illusions and hallucinations, are common. In addition to alterations in mental status and behavior, tremor, dysarthria, ataxia, asterixis, multifocal myoclonus, and autonomic dysfunction including fever, tachycardia, and hypertension can be seen.

Although almost any complicating illness may bring out a confusional state in an elderly person. The most common are febrile infectious diseases, especially cases that resist the effect of antibiotic medication; trauma, concussive brain injuries; surgical operations, particularly those requiring large amounts of anesthesia and pre and postoperative medication; and congestive heart failure, chronic respiratory disease, and severe anemia, especially pernicious anemia.

Amnestic Disorders. This disorder is characterized by memory impairment in the absence of other significant cognitive impairments. The single symptom of a memory disturbance causes significant impairment in social or occupational functioning. There is impairment in the ability to learn new information (anterograde amnesia) and the inability to recall previously remembered knowledge (retrograde amnesia).

Psychogenic amnesia is characterized by the sudden inability to recall important personal information. This failure of memory can take several forms: (a) generalized amnesia, which spans all previous life experiences; (b) continuous amnesia, which encompasses the time period following a particular event up to and including the present; (c) localized amnesia, in which there is a failure to recall all events that took place during a particular period of time: (d) selective amnesia, characterized by patchy memory failure for some events but not others within circumscribed period of time. In all types, the patient's sensorium is clear, although there may be perplexity and disorientation. Onset and recovery are usually complete. The diagnosis of amnestic disorder cannot be made when a patient has other signs of cognitive impairment, such as those seen in dementia, or when a patient has impaired attention or consciousness, such as that seen in delirium.

Brain Tumors. The most common initial manifestations of brain tumors are headache and seizures. The headache may be worse in the morning or may awaken the patient at night. It may correlate in location with the site of the tumor or may be diffuse. Seizures can be focal or generalized and may begin as absence attacks that are initially ignored by the patient.

Focal signs include homonymous hemianopia (temporal lesion), ataxia (cerebellar lesion), Parinaud's syndrome (paralysis of conjugate upward gaze from lesions in the pineal-superior colliculus area), and Nothnagel's syndrome (staggering, oculomotor paralysis, and nystagmus from midbrain tumors). Examples of false localized signs include upgoing toes on the same side as the tumor because of compression of the opposite cerebral peduncle against the tentorium and cerebellar dysfunction resulting from compression of the cerebellum by tumors located in the cerebrum.

Less common non-focal symptoms include personality changes, nausea, speech and visual disturbances, and decreased level of consciousness. Brain edema is a most important aspect of tumor growth, but it also assumes importance in cerebral trauma, infarction, abscess, and hypoxia-as well as in certain toxic and metabolic states (see Table 10-4).

Table 10-4. Lesions that alter the blood brain barrier

Brain Edema	Features of Cerebral Neoplasms
Vasogenic Edema	Tumor growths as well as in toxic injury to the blood vessels that is limited to the white matter
Cytotoxic Edema	Occurs with hypoxic injury in which cellular elements (neurons, glia, and endothelial cells) Imbibe fluid and swell
Cellular Edema	It may complicate acute hypo-osmolality of the plasma, as occurs with dilutional hyponatremia, inappropriate secretion of antidiuretic hormone, or an osmotic disequilibrium syndrome.
Interstitial (hydrocephalic edema)	It extends for only 2 to 3 mm from the ventricular wall in association with tension hydrocephalus.

Stroke Syndromes. Due to the blockages, the brain is deprived of blood and the vital oxygen carried by the blood. Interruption of blood flow for 30 seconds or more impairs cerebral function. If there is a total loss of oxygen for more than 5 minutes, irreversible damage will occur. The seriousness of a stroke depends on whether a given area of the brain has alternate supplies of blood available which can circumvent the area that is partially or totally occluded. Damage to the brain occurs not only from a loss of oxygen and the blood supply but also from the toxic effect of the blood on the brain tissue and the resulting swelling of the brain.

Diagnostic criteria that are used to describe cerebrovascular disease include:

- Transient ischemic attacks (TIA): Transient neurologic symptoms that usually last not more than 15 minutes, but by arbitrary definition can last up to 24 hours.
- Reversible Ischemic neurologic deficit (RIND); the deficit persists more than 24 hours, but resolves in several days.
- Progressive stroke or stroke-in-evolution: A neurologic impairment that progresses over hours or a day or two.

Patients who have had a recent hemorrhagic stroke may be at risk for rebleeding during ECT. Withholding ECT for a period of weeks to months is recommended if the patient has had a stroke. However, this delay must be weighed against the severity of the psychiatric illness itself. Extremes of blood pressure, both hyper- and hypotension, should be avoided during ECT in stroke patients. (see Table 10-5). The use of intravenous anti-hypertensives during ECT may be helpful in some cases. Less definite risk factors include cigarette smoking, obesity, high plasma fibrinogen, excessive alcohol consumption, and hyperlipidemia.

Table 10-5. Localization of Intracerebral Hemorrhages

SITE OF HEMORRHAGE   NEUROLOGIC SYMPTOMS

Putaminal Hemorrhage	The most common syndrome when patients lapse almost immediately into stupor and coma with hemiplegia; The face sags on one side, speech becomes slurred or aphasic, the arm and leg gradually weaken, and the eyes tend to deviate away from the side of the paretic limbs.
Thalamic Hemorrhage	Sensory deficit equals or exceeds the motor weakness. Aphasia with lesions of the dominant side. A series of ocular disturbances: palsies of vertical and lateral gaze, forced deviation of the eyes downward, inequality of pupils with absence of light reaction, skew deviation with the eye opposite the hemorrhage being displaced downward and medially, ipsilateral ptosis and miosis, and retraction nystagmus.
Pontine Hemorrhage	Deep coma ensues in a few minutes. Total paralysis, decerebrate rigidity, and small pupils that react to light. Lateral movements, crossed sensory or motor disturbances, and cranial nerve palsies.

Cerebellar Hemorrhage	Repeated vomiting. Occipital headache, vertigo, and inability to sit, stand, or walk. Conjugate lateral gaze to the side of the hemorrhage, forced deviation of the eyes to the opposite side, or an ipsilateral sixth nerve weakness. Ocular signs include blepharospasm, involuntary closure of one eye, skew deviation, and samall, unequal pupils.
Lobar Hemorrhage	In the occipital lobe pain occurs around the ipsilateral eye and a dense homonymous hemianopia. In the temporal lobe, pain anterior to the ear, partial hemianopia, and fluent aphasia. In the frontal lobe contralateral hemiplegia, mainly of the arm, and frontal headache. In the parietal lobe anterior temporal headache and hemi-sensory deficit contralaterally occur.

Epilepsy. In epilepsy, the grand mal seizure often begins with a sudden loss of consciousness and fall to the ground. The initial motor signs are a brief flexion of the trunk, an opening of the mouth and eyelids, and upward deviation of the eyes. The arms are elevated and abducted, the elbows semiflexed, and the hands pronated. These are followed by a more protracted extension phase, involving first the back and neck, then the arms and legs. There may be piercing cry as the whole musculature is seized in a spasm and air is forcibly emitted through the closed vocal cords. Since the respiratory muscles are caught up in the tonic spasm, breathing is suspended, and after some seconds, the skin and mucous membranes become cyanotic. The pupils are dilated and unreactive to light. The bladder may empty at this stage or later, during the postictal coma. This is the tonic phase of the seizure and lasts for 10 to 20 seconds.

In contrast to major generalized seizures, absence (petit mal) seizures are notable for their brevity and the paucity of motor activity. They may be so brief that the patients resemble a moment of absent-mindedness or daydreaming. Automatisms, in the form of up smacking, chewing, and fumbling movements of the fingers, are common during an attack. As a rule, such patients do not fall, and they may even continue such complex acts as walking or riding a bicycle.

Depression is common in epilepsy. Among epileptic patients, those with partial complex seizures have the highest suicide rate. Hypochondriacal features, agitation, and suspiciousness or frank paranoia often accompany depression in the elderly. Major depression in the elderly often requires pharmacotherapy or electroconvulsive therapy.

The most theoretically interesting use of ECT in neurologic illness is for the treatment of epilepsy. The effects of ECT on seizure threshold have led to an understanding of the potent anticonvulsant properties of ECT. Many aspects of ECT's anticonvulsant properties need to be worked out before such an application would be feasible. For example, for what seizure type would ECT be most effective: partial or generalized? Would ECT effectively interrupt status epilepticus? What electrode placement and electrical dosing strategy would be optimal? What interval between maintenance treatments would be necessary to provide adequate protection against seizures?

Deborah Y. Liggan, MD

10.2 Cardiovascular Diseases

The goal of treating hypertension is to reduce the risk of morbidity and mortality due to the cardiovascular consequences of the disorder. The initial therapy of hypertension should be directed at non-pharmacologic alterations in the patient's lifestyle. Such therapy should include dietary modifications to reduce sodium, alcohol, and caffeine intake. Weight reduction should be recommended to the obese individual. Exercise should be encouraged and behavior modification should be considered to reduce stressful lifestyles.

Patients with pre-existing hypertension may have a greater increase in blood pressure during ECT than patients without pre-existing hypertension. For patients who escape control during ECT with pressures in excess of 220 mmHg systolic or 120 mmHg diastolic, administration of esmol or labetalol will usually suffice, although augmentation with nifedipine may be necessary.

The principle of physiologic stress during ECT is the autonomic sympathetic stimulus to the heart and the peripheral vasculature. Ictal electrocardiogram changes may include peaked T waves, ST-segment depression, ventricular ectopy, and even runs of ventricular tachycardia. In the addition there is an immediate rise in cardiac contractility and peripheral vascular tone, resulting in immediate rises in systolic and diastolic blood pressure and cardiac rate.

Complete evaluation of the cardiovascular system extends beyond the examination of the heart itself. Cardiovascular risk factors I the medically ill elderly include hypertension, myocardial infarction, cardiac arrhythmias, and congestive heart failure. (Drop +Welch 1989).

Hypertension is typically classified as mild, moderate, or severe, depending upon the level of the diastolic blood pressure. The prevalence of hypertension also increases with advancing age. The basic preoperative evaluation in the hypertensive patient should establish whether there is end-organ damage (renal: serum creatinine concentration and urinalysis; cerebrovascular: history, neurologic and neurovascular examination; and cardiovascular: history, cardiac examination, chest x-ray, and electro cardiogram).

Hypertenison can be very damaging because of two primary effect: (1) increased work load on the heart and (2) damage to the arteries by the excessive pressure. Cardiac muscle, like skeletal muscle, hypertrophies when its work load increases. In hypertension, the very high pressure against which the left ventricle mist beat causes it to increase in weight as much as two to threefold. Therefore, relative ischemia of the left ventricle develops as the hypertension becomes more and more severe. In the late stages of hypertension this can become serious enough that the person develops angina pectoris.

Physiologic principles indicate that pressure is a direct function of flow and resistance. The blood pressure, therefore, is related to the cardiac output and the peripheral vascular resistance. High pressure in the arteries not only causes coronary sclerosis but also sclerosis of blood vessels throughout all the remainder of the body.

Myocardial Infarction. Tachycardia; pallor; small arterial pulse; narrow pulse pressure; apical late systolic bulge of ischemic myocardium; soft heart sounds; presystolic or early diastolic extra sounds; pericardial friction rub; apical systolic murmur (papillary muscle dysfunction); any of the arrhythmias.

Patients with recent myocardial infarction should not be automatically excluded from ECT, and the risks of treatment should be weighed against the potential lethality of remaining depressed. Evaluation begins with a thorough assessment of cardiac function. The four parameters of interest are supply, contractility, and stress tolerance.

Cardiac Arrhythmias. There are three basic causes of disturbance in the rhythm of the heart: suppression or enhancement of initiation or propagation of the action potential, reentry of the action potential into a pathway through which it has already passed, and triggered activity. More than one of these mechanisms may be operative in producing a particular arrhythmia. Abnormal slowing of the heart rate produces bradyarrhythmia, and if there is rapid sustained firing of the ectopic focus, a tachyarrhythmia ensues.

Arrhythmias may or may not cause symptoms. These symptoms are caused by an appreciation of the irregular rhythm (palpitations) or by a reduction in cardiac output (light-headedness, dizziness, presyncope, syncope, dyspnea, diaphoresis, chest pain, and anxiety) especially in the elderly.

When taking a history from a patient with a suspected arrhythmia, it is important to define the onset, regularity, and duration of symptoms, and whether any factors seem to trigger symptoms (e.g. smoking, drinking coffee, exercise, emotional stress, and taking or forgetting to take medications). It is important to determine whether there is a history or symptoms of an underlying disease that may be associated with arrhythmia. This includes hypertension, heart failure, ischemic or valvular heart disease, and thyrotoxicosis.

Most cardiac arrhythmias are manageable once they have been correctly diagnosed. ECT may unmask latent ventricular arrhythmias that can become much more evident during the course of treatment. In addition, of the conduction defects, first degree heart block may be rapidly progressive and insertion of a cardiac pacemaker may be necessary before ECT.

Congestive Heart Failure. The prevalence of heart failure increases greatly in patients over 60 years old and is at least 25% greater among the African-American population than among the white population. Over the age of 70, women with congestive heart failure outnumber men.

Heart failure is caused by one of three basic mechanisms: an increased work load of which the heart cannot accommodate, a disorder of the myocardium so that it is unable to accommodate normal work loads, or a restriction of ventricular filling so that an adequate stroke volume cannot be achieved. The most common symptoms of heart failure are dyspnea and fatigue. Dyspnea in heart failure is a symptom of increased left ventricular end-diastolic pressure with pulmonary venous and capillary congestion. Increased pulmonary congestion causes decreased lung compliance and vital capacity. The work of breathing increases and breathing becomes rapid, shallow, and forced. Fatigue, caused by low cardiac output, is often described as a general sense of weakness or lack of ambition. Some patients may complain of fatigue rather than dyspnea. The ejection fraction should be determined, because patients with an ejection fraction of less than 20% are at risk for transient pulmonary edema during ECT. In addition, patients who are given oxygen and furosemide will usually recompensate within 15-30 minutes.

10.3 Pulmonary Diseases

Obstructive lung diseases are the most common forms of chronic pulmonary disease encountered in ambulatory practice. The diagnosis, severity, clinical course, and response to treatment can best be established by objective tests of lung function. For example, obstructive lung diseases cause the lung to empty slowly during a forced expiratory maneuver. Normal people can forcefully expel all of the air that can leave their lungs (the vital capacity) within 4 to 6 seconds. And people with established obstructive lung disease may continue to expire during a forced expiratory maneuver for 10 to 20 seconds or more.

Asthma is a disorder characterized symptomatically by cough, chest tightness, shortness of breath, and wheezing associated with limitation of airflow (according to the vital capacity). The symptoms may be acute and episodic or may wax and wane over long periods. One or more of the symptoms may be dominant, but usually all are present. The airflow obstruction is a variable and usually, although not always, returns to the normal range between exacerbations. Between episodes, most asthmatics are symptom free, but they are susceptible to attacks of wheezing, cough, and chest tightness when exposed to various triggers. It is important to note that inflammation of the airways and bronchial hyperactivity are nearly universally found in asthmatics.

The goals of the treatment of asthma are to keep the patient symptom free day and night, with full activity levels, normal lung function, absent side effects, and satisfaction with the process of care. Treatment in the ambulatory setting has four major components: monitoring of symptoms and lung function, control of environmental triggers, education of the patient and family, and drug therapy. Both patients and physicians should understand that untreated severe asthma can be fatal and should recognize the individual at risk.

Whenever possible, the theophylline dosage should be decreased or discontinued before ECT because it lowers the seizure threshold and may be a cause of partial ictal activity or even status epilepticus after ECT. If it is necessary for pulmonary management, then patients should be observed for post-treatment seizure activity for several hours after treatment.

Pneumonia may be defined as infection of the pulmonary parenchyma. Clinically the acute onset of cough, sputum production, pleuritic chest pain, fever, and chills together with a new pulmonary infiltrate on chest radiograph are consistent with the diagnosis of pneumonia. There are forms of pneumonitis other than those caused by infection, particularly chemical pneumonitis resulting from aspiration of gastric acid or exposure to an exogenous irritant.

As the percentage of the general population above 65 years of age rises, so does the importance of early diagnosis and treatment of pneumonia. Studies of pneumonia in the elderly have indicated that they have a higher mortality and a greater chance of progression of disease despite treatment. Management of the patient with pneumonia involves stabilization and general supportive care as well as specific antibiotic treatment directed at the most likely etiologic agent. If a patient develops pneumonia during a course of ECT, that is a warning that the protocol for recovery from general anesthesia may be in need of review.

Chronic Obstructive Pulmonary Disease (COPD) refers to a group of disorders that have slowly progressive airways obstruction. The course of the disease is punctuated by periodic exacerbations resulting in an increase in dyspnea and sputum production or occasionally, the precipitation of acute respiratory failure. These exacerbations are often due to pulmonary infection, the development of heart failure, or poor patient compliance with prescribed therapy. In COPD, patients usually present with dyspnea and exercise intolerance. Physical examination reveals signs of lung overinflation, prominent use of accessory respiratory muscles, diminished breath sounds, and diffuse wheezing especially during a forced expiration.

Three pathophysiologic disorders are recognized as a part of the syndrome of COPD: emphysema, small airways disease, and chronic bronchitis.

Emphysema is characterized by two features. Anatomically, it is defined as an abnormal enlargement of the air spaces distal to the terminal bronchioles, accompanied by destructive changes in the alveolar walls. Physiologically, it is characterized by a loss of elastic recoil and thus an increased lung compliance.

In **Small Airways Disease** the earliest manifestation of COPD appears to be in the peripheral airways. Abnormalities that have been identified include inflammation of the terminal and respiratory bronchioles, fibrosis of the airway walls leading to narrowing, and goblet cell metaplasia. These lesions contribute to airways obstruction, although the correlation is not as close as with the degree emphysema.

Chronic Bronchitis is defined as a persistent cough resulting in sputum production for more than 3 months in each year over the previous 3 years. The airways obstruction seen in the setting of chronic bronchitis is due to associated emphysema, bronchospasm, and obstruction of the peripheral airways.

10.4 Endocrine Diseases

Endocrine glands play dominant roles in our lives. Dysfunction in any endocrine gland has consequences. The products of the glands control life's cycles, from daily feeding and sleeping, growth and maturation, sex and fetal development, to senescene and death. Seizures most commonly occur after an acute change in endocrine function and usually result from electrolyte imbalance.

Diabetes Mellitus is characterized by an abnormal increase in the concentration of blood glucose. The most common varieties of diabetes are known to be associated with abnormalities of insulin secretion and concentration, cellular resistance to insulin action, and the development after many years of vascular damage to various organs, especially the kidneys, eyes, cardiovascular system, and nervous system.

Type I diabetes is a chronic autoimmune disease, characterized by destruction of beta cells in pancreatic islets and by failure of those cells to synthesize insulin.

Type II diabetes is the most common form of diabetes mellitus and accounts for approximately 80% to 90% of patients presenting with an abnormality of glucose metabolism. These patients are ordinarily neither absolutely dependent on treatment with insulin nor ketosis prone. Nonetheless, patients being treated with oral hypoglycemic drugs may require insulin to control hyperglycemia or ketoacidosis during stress. Behavioral and possibly environment factors appear to be involved in the onset of type 2 diabetes. Especially prominent is the role of excessive caloric intake and subsequent obesity in 60% to 90% of cases (See Table 10-6). Each diabetic patient should undergo comprehensive preoperative evaluation. Most diabetic patients can undergo outpatient surgery if their diabetes is stable, whether controlled by diet alone, oral agents, or insulin. Additionally, approximately 14% of diabetic patients have postoperative complications that may be related to diabetes, particularly wound infection (See Table 10-7).

Table 10-6. Comparison of Type I and Type II Diabetes

	Type I	Type II
Synonym Age of onset Ketosis Body Weight	IDDM Juvenile onset Common Non-obese	NIDDM Adult onset Uncommon Obese (50-90%)
Endogenous Insulin Secretion	Severe Deficiency	Moderate Deficiency
Insulin Resistance	Occasional	Almost Always
HLA association	DR3, DR4	None
Islet cell antibodies	Frequent	Absent
Association with other autoimmune disease	Frequent	No
Treatment with Insulin	Always necessary	Usually not required

Table 10-7. Chronic Complications of Diabetes

Microvascular Disease

- Retinopathy
- Nephropathy

Macrovacular Disease

- Coronary Artery Disease
- Cerbrovacular Disease
- Peripheral Vacular Disease

Neuropathic

- Peripheral Symmetric Polyneuropathy
- Mononeuropathies
- Autonomic Neuropathies
- Diabetic Amyotrophy

Foot Ulcers

Dermopathies

Infections

- Gingival
- Dermal
- Vulvovaginal

Cushing's Syndrome. The consequence of chronic exposure to excessive amounts of glucocorticoid hormone, Cushing's Syndrome occurs as a consequence of increased endogenous production of cortisol, or more commonly, as the result of prolonged exposure to glucocorticoids administered exogenously in superphysiologic doses.

In Cushing's disease, the hypersecretion of adrenocorticotropin (ACTH), by the pituitary gland is due to the presence of an adenoma in approximately 90% of cases. This disorder is much more common in women (female – male ratio, 5:1), typically occurs during the childbearing years, and as a consequence of an insidious onset, may go undetected for many years.

The clinical manifestations of Cushing's disease are very diverse. Regardless of the etiology, hypercortisolism results in obesity, carbohydrate intolerance, muscle wasting and osteoporosis. Obesity is centripetal, manifested typically by a buffalo hump, increased supraclavicular fat pads, and moon facies. Easy bruise ability and abdominal striae may be noted. Mild hypertension is common. Depression occurs often, and rarely patients may be frankly psychotic. An increase in adrenal androgen production can result in hirsutism, acne, and menstrual disorders in women. Men may complain of impotence and loss of libido. Treatment of Cushing's Syndrome depends on its cause. Pituitary microsurgery employing the transsphenoidal approach is now the treatment of choice for patients with suspected pituitary adenomas. In experienced hands, and an adenoma may be localized in 90 per cent of patients and removed with a low morbidity. This approach has the advantage of preserving the surrounding pituitary tissue, so that hypopituitarism is a rare complication.

Addison's Disease. This classical form of adrenal insufficiency, described by Addison, is due to primary disease of the adrenals. It is characterized by pigmentation of the skin and mucous membranes; nausea, vomiting, and weight loss; and muscle weakness, languor, and a tendency to faint. Since Addison's time, hypotension, hyperkalemia, hyponatremia, and low serum cortisol concentrations have come to be recognized as important clinical features. Mental changes include irritability, confusion, disorientation, and convulsions, with or without hypoglycemia. Some of these mental abnormalities are related to the disturbances of electrolyte balance. The fatigue in adrenal insufficiency is usually absent when the patient awakens in the morning and becomes progressively severe with activity during the day. This is in contra distinction to patients with functional neurasthenia, who complain of feeling just as tired upon awakening as when going to bed. Adrenal insufficiency of whatever cause is a life-threatening condition; there is always a danger of collapse and even death, particularly during periods of infection, surgery, or injury.

Thyroid Disorders. Dysfunction of the thyroid gland causes some of the most common endocrine disorders. Thyrotoxicosis (hyperthyroidism) is a consequence of excess thyroid hormone. Graves' disease is the most common cause of thyrotoxicosis. The patient most frequently presents with a history of nervousness, heat intolerance, sweating, palpitations, tremor, and weight loss. In addition, a change in collar size (goiter formation) and eye discomfort (Grave's opthalmopathy) maybe noted. Skeletal muscle wasting, especially of the limb girdles may cause patients to experience difficulty in climbing stairs or getting up from the sitting position. The mental and emotional changes include anxiety, irritability, poor concentration, restlessnesss, emotional lability, and insomnia, especially in the elderly. A deficiency of thyroid hormone causes hypothyroidism (myxedema). In this condition the patient may feel puffy and complain of continual coldness. He may note dry skin, hoarsening and deepening of the voice, thinning and increased brittleness of the hair, fatigue, slowing of thought and movement and chronic constipation. Seizures may be presenting sign in 20% of all hypothyroid patients, and are nearly always generalized. When overt psychosis occurs, it is defined as myxedema madness. Thyroid dysfunction is frequently manifested clinically by a swelling (enlargement) of the gland, a condition referred to as goiter formation. Iodine, a substrate for thyroid hormone synthesis, also plays an auto-regulatory role in the metabolism of the thyroid gla

10.5 Self-Assessment Questions

1. How do the dopamine –enhancing effects of ECT relate to the treatment of Parkinson's disease?

2. What cognitive function presents when dementia coexisits with depression?

3. What four parameters are used in the assessment of cardiac function before ECT?

4. Identify three measures which are used in the assessment of congestive heart failure.

5. What symptoms of poor dentition present in elderly patients who are at high risk for dental fracture with ECT?

6. How are meds and strategies necessary for pulmonary management with ECT?

7. What clinical features define Addison's disease?

8. What subjective depressive symptoms are difficult for expression in patients with dementia?

9. Identify the clinical features that present with Parkinson's Disease that render it a public health issue.

10. Describe the use of ECT in neurologic illness as it is used for the treatment of epilepsy.

Chapter One: The History of ECT

Reference Notes

1) Early Romans put curative powers in the seizures of epileptics to treat head pain by generating an electric pulse potent enough to produce a convulsion.

2) The theory was: the more severe the convulsion, the better the results. These early patients often let out a shriek as the electricity was applied, but as they convulsed, they blacked out.

3) Chemically induced seizures were used to treat:

   - Dementia praecox (schizophrenia)
   - Major depressions
   - Intractable mania

4) A successful method was designed in Rome by Ugo Cerletti and Lucio Bini, where alternating current form a wall socket from positive to negative at 45 hertz, calling this form of current a sine wave.

5) In the mid 1950's, Dr. Max Fink described the effects of both psychotropic drugs and ECT on the electroencephograph (EEG), which recorded overall patterns of brain activity to ensure that a proper grand mal seizure had occurred.

6) ECT is known to enhance dopaminergic, serotonergic, and adrenergic neurotransmission.

7) The primary contributor to the impedance of the electrical circuit is not the brain, but rather the skin, the underlying scalp soft tissues, and the skull.

8) Common medical conditions in which ECT was used to treat patients with remarkable effect:

Chronic obstructive pulmonary Disease (COPD)
   Asthma
   Hypertension
   Coronary Artery Disease
History of myocardial infarction
Cardiac Arrhythmia
History of Cerebrovascular Accident
Osteoporosis

9) A professional trained in anesthesia is a required member of the ECT treatment team. Brief, light general anesthesia is used during ECT to achieve amnesia and absence of pain for the procedure. In addition, muscular relaxation is used during ECT t eliminate musculoskeletal injury and to aid in airway management.

10) Under the influence of Harold Sackeim, a professor of psychiatry at Columbia Psychiatric Institute, it became the norm to limit the amount of electricity used to dose only marginally in excess of the seizure threshold.

Chapter Two: Madness Curd with Electricity

Reference Notes

1) Basing their views on Freudian theory, researchers imagined that seizures suppressed memories of childhood trauma that they deemed to be the basis for psychological symptoms.

2) Serum cortisol is increased after ECT in the postictal period. The observed decrease in baseline and postictal cortisol levels during a course of ECT is nonspecific and may be caused by a reduction of depression-related stress. The plasma cortisol response to ECT is dose-dependent.

3) The serotonin system is the only monoaminergic system in which ECT is believed to have opposite effects from most antidepressant drugs.

4) Corroboration of a grand mal seizure comes from three sources:

   a) An electrocardiogram that shows a spike in heart rate
   b) An electroencephalogram that reveals changes in the brain's electrical activity
   c) A blood pressure cuff that reflects an increase in pressures.

5) The Hippocratic axon "premium non nocere" (above all, do no harm), which combines the principles of beneficence and non-maleficence: "I will use treatment to help the sick according to my ability and judgment, but I will never use it to injure or wrong them."

6) Insulin causes the liver and muscles to remove circulating glucose form the blood, which means denying it as well to the brain. In the absence of glucose the brain goes into a coma or stupor, which is called "insulin shock." With additional insulin injections, he displayed tonic-clinic convulsions and biting his tongue. After the seizure, the patient had complete amnesia for the preceding events, and his memory loss lasted an hour and a half.

7) ECT starts working in one to two weeks, versus medication therapies that can take six to eight weeks. This is significant because the faster that a treatment works, the sooner patients can start rebuilding their lives.

8) According to medical statics, suicide does not work for alcoholics because they have a high seizure threshold and often are unresponsive to the ECT.

9) Metrazol convulsion therapy was superior to insulin coma therapy because it was safer-patients in deep coma were often at the brink of death. The essential factor in Metrazol therapy was the convulsion, whereas in insulin coma the agent was hypoglycemia. Metrazol's appeal in the U.S. was its efficacy in mood disorders. Depression was considered unresponsive to insulin.

10) ECT does not cause brain damage, change personality, or turn the patient into Frankenstein's relative. It also does not affect metabolism, heart, weight, appetite, sex drive, sexual performance, cause dry mouth, vomiting, diarrhea, life-threatening rash, or any other common or bizarre side effects. Instead, studies show that the side effects of ECT are generally headaches and temporary memory loss.

Chapter Three: Patient Preparation

Reference Notes

1) Laboratory evaluation:

   - Electrocardiogram
   - Complete blood count
   - Electrolytes
   - Liver function tests
   - Other tests specific to patient's medical condition

2) Most diabetic patients are more stable if the morning dose of insulin is held until after their treatment. The insulin requirement usually decreases as a diabetic patient recovers from depression, and blood glucose levels must be monitored frequently during the course of ECT.

3) The inability to carry out purposeful movements on command, in the absence of problems of comprehension, muscular strength, or coordination is a motor apraxia and indicates brain dysfunction.

4) When the patient is laid down on the treatment bed and has an intravenous line, he receives a short-acting muscle relaxant, succinylcholine is administered.

5) The design of informed consent came to a head in 1966, by Henry Beecher, a professor of anesthesiology at Harvard University, in a New England Journal of Medicine article.

6) As coded in AB 4481, ECT could be given only after

   a) The patient gives written informed consent

b) The patient has the capacity to consent

c) A relative has been given a thorough oral explanation

d) All other treatments have been exhausted and the treatment is critically needed

e) There has been a review by three appointed physicians who agree with the treating physician that the patient has the capacity to consent

7) Even though a patient voluntarily signs an agreement to receive ECT, he may withdraw his consent at any time, even before the first treatment is given or whether the patient's continued treatment is the best alternative methods available.

8) A strategy for seizure prolongation is the intravenous administration of caffeine 5 minutes before ECT.

9) Atropine remains the drug of choice for attenuating or blocking the direct vagal effects on the heart during and immediately after the passage of the electrical stimulus and in the immediate postictal period.

10) Patients with coronary artery disease may be pretreated with 1 inch of nitroglycerin paste applied to the chest or one sublingual squirt of nitroglycerin spray at least 30 minutes before ECT.

Chapter Four: Treatment Procedure

Reference Notes

1) Systemic changes that may occur during ECT include:

   - A brief episode of hypotension and bradycardia
   - followed by sinus tachycardia
   - sympathetic hyperactivity
   - An increase in blood pressure

2) The most important reason to monitor the EEG during ECT is to assure that the seizure ends completely, because paroxysmal brain electrical activity commonly continues after motor activity has ended.

3) ECT devices differ in terms of the typeof electrical stimulus that is actually delivered to the patient, with perhaps the most important distinction being that of waveform (sinusoidal versus brief pulse).

4) Succinylcholine is given to block this drug from the muscles distal to the cuff and permit safe observation of the unmodified seizure.

5) Self-stick ECG recording electrodes are applied precordially above and below the heart, with a third applied to the shoulder as a ground. The appropriate ECG leads are then connected and a baseline rhythm strip is obtained.

6) Thenon (1956) was the first to demonstrate the specific link between right unilateral electrode placement and reduced memory loss and confusion.

7) Methohexital has become the standard anesthetic for ECT because it has rapid onset, has brief duration, and causes minimal post-anesthesia confusion.

8) In the first (depolarization) phase of succinylcholine will appear first in the muscles of the head, next, and upper chest and spread to those of the trunk and limbs before reaching the small muscles of the feet and hands. When the fasciculations have died down in the small muscles of the feet (generally about one minute after the succinylcholine injection), the patient is ready to be treated.

9) Seizure threshold is the minimum amount of electricity needed to induce a seizure.

10) The tonic and clinic muscle contractions measure the efficacy by a rise in the serum level of prolactin, a peptide released into the blood with a seizure.

Chapter Five: Postictal Care

Reference Notes

1) Approximately 10% of patients will develop marked agitation and restlessness immediately postictally. This event is easily managed with a short-acting, rapid-onset benzodiazepine administered intravenously.

2) The brain has a period of quiescence in which it becomes quiet, and its natural activity rests and recovers. It's also typical for patients to feel sleepy, not remember events surrounding the seizure, and even possibly suffer disorientation.

3) Common factors contributing to the short seizure lasting less than 20 seconds:

   - Excessive anesthetic dose
   - A concurrent anticonvulsant, or another with anticonvulsant properties, such as a benzodiazepine or lidocaine
   - Lack of good hyperventilation
   - Inadequate electrical stimulus dose

4) Steps that should be taken in the case of a prolonged seizure lasting more than 2 or 3 minutes:

   - Administer an anticonvulsant. Give 50% of the dose or an intravenous benzodiazepine.
   - Continue to oxygenate (but not hyperventilate) while watching the EEG for cessation of epileptiform activity.
   - If after 1-2 minutes the seizure is still ongoing, repeat the medication given above.
   - Continue pharmacological interventions along with full medical support of the patient until seizure activity is ended.

5) ECT affects memory and cognition in three ways:

- An acute postictal confusional state. This side effect is much more severe with bilateral ECT than with right unilateral ECT, and it may be more prolonged in elderly patients.
- Anterograde memory dysfunction
- Retrograde memory dysfunction

6) Concentrating the seizure in the prefrontal cortex, the site of higher thinking, is the best way to ensure that it is maximally effect.

7) The side effect of headache following ECT, may be related to the contraction of the temporalis and masseter muscles or to the cerebral hemodynamic changes that accompany the treatment.

8) Nausea may be treated with 6.25—25.0mg promethazine intramuscularly, before or immediately after ECT, before the patient awakens. Nausea may also be prevented by anticholinergic premedication.

9) The patient and the post-ECT caretaker are advised that the patient should refrain from engaging in any activity that requires a high level of concentration or judgement, such as driving a car or operating machinery, for the rest of the day.

10) After treatment, patients should always be rolled on their side to prevent aspiration of secretions and obstruction of the airway. There should be a staff member whose sole responsibility is to monitor the respirations and vital signs of recovering patients and prevent injury due to post-treatment agitation.

Chapter Six: The Self-Vignette

Reference Notes

1) Affective disorders associated with the highest success with ECT:

   - Major depressive episode (unipolar and bipolar)
   - Mania
   - Mixed affective state
   - Catatonia
   - Schizophrenia with prominent affective symptoms
   - Schizoaffective disorder

2) Steps taken to make the home environment safe:

   1. Have no guns at home
   2. Take medicines as prescribed and not over take them or under take them
   3. Do not drive an auto
   4. Review the Safety Plan and keep it available for easy access in a time of crisis

3) Younger patients typically recover fully and quickly. Older patients have longer recovery times, and their families often see them drowsy and confused. These experiences are disturbing to patients, their families, nurses, and caretakers and contribute to the popular notion that memory is severely affected by the treatment.

4) Three broad domains characterize depression:

   - Disorders of mood
   - Cognitive function
   - Neurovegetative function

5) In right-handed individuals, the center for the control of speech and for memory is almost always on the left-side of the brain, the dominant side. In left-handed individuals, the speech center is usually on the right-side. Delivery on the nondominat side lessens the effects on memory. Since dominance for speech and memory lies in the left hemisphere in more than 95 percent of the population, the unilateral electrodes are usually placed on the right side; this is unilateral nondominant ECT.

6) An example is the increase in prolactin, a product of the pituitary gland which peaks 20 to 40 munutes after a seizure as evidence that a grand mal brain seizure has taken place.

7) Patients are sleepless, appetite is poor, and weight loss may be pronounced, at times amounting to 20% of the body weight within a few weeks. Work, sexual activity, and family may be disregarded. The future appears hopeless, patients believe they are helpless to affect it, and their thoughts are filled with gloom.

8) Benzodiazepines may decrease the intensity or generalization of the ECT seizure. They may also shorten seizure duration, and their use may increase the number of ECT treatments required for recovery. The authors recommended discontinuing benzodiazepines before unilateral ECT is given.

9) Seizure threshold is the minimum amount of electricity needed to induce a seizure. What factors increase the seizure threshold? These include the patient's age, sex, and laterality of electrode placement. This method provides only an educated guess about the patient's true threshold and is therefore less accurate than empirical seizure threshold determination.

10) A professional trained in anesthesia is a required member of the ECT treatment team. The primary goals are patient safety and comfort. Brief, light general anesthesia is used during ECT to achieve amnesia and absence of pain for the procedure. Muscular relaxation is used during ECT to eliminate musculoskeletal injury and to aid in airway management. The patient receives supplemental oxygen, usually 100% O2 via mask, throughout the procedure.

Chapter Seven: ECT Discussion

Reference Notes

1) Patients need medications that are faster acting than antidepressants, which can take weeks to kick in. Consider treatment with ECT generally starts working within a couple of sessions, meaning couple of days.

2) Congestive heart failure is usually treatable with oxygen and elevation of the head. Sometimes it becomes necessary to treat with intravenous furosemide and morphine.

3) The vascular depression hypothesis posits that vascular lesions in white matter disrupt key pathways, leading to a disconnection syndrome with abnormal functional activation in downstream cortical and limbic regions and resulting in impaired mood regulation, cognition, and neurovegetative function.

4) For the elderly, ECT's very success in treating depression can unlock hidden dementia. Major depression is also the commonest cause of reversible dementia, and a successful ECT treatment that can lift the dementia along with the depression.

5) Explain how the heart is physiologically stressed during ECT:

   - Cardiac work increases abruptly at the onset of the seizure initially because of sympathetic outflow from the diencephalon, through the spinal sympathetic tract, to the heart.

- This outflow is augmented by a rise in circulating catecholamine levels that peak about 3 minutes after the onset of seizure activity.
- After the seizure ends, parasympathetic tone remains strong, often causing transient bradycardia and hypotension, with a return to baseline function in 5 to 10 minutes.

6) Behaviors for which ECT is ineffective:

- Severe character pathology
- Substance abuse and dependence
- Sexual identification disorders
- Psychoneuroses
- Chronicity of illness without flagrant psychopathology

7) Psychoneuroses that demonstrate clinical symptoms ineffective for ECT:

- Hysterical disorder
- Briquete's syndrome
- Hypochondriasis
- Panic or anxiety disorders
- Pain syndromes
- Obsessive-compulsive disorders

8) The most common, persistent, and hotly debated effect, called retrograde amnesia, involves the loss of memories starting around the time ECT is given and extending back months or even years.

9) Frequent and fundamental questions that face ECT physicians because of the procedure's risks:

- Whether the information they give potential patients adequately reflects the procedure's risks
- Are consent forms used by ECT doctors
- Is a model offered today in which standard with any surgery and should be with any psychotropic drug

10) Brain damage reflected in the front line in the battle between ECT's boosters and detractors, both sides increasingly are resorted to regard actions that impugn the other's motives and underline its conflicts of interest.

Chapter Eight: Geriatric Psychiatry

Reference Notes

1) Changes that occur with hearing impairment due to aging: a decline in high frequency speech perception and auditory discrimination. Hearing impairment may lead to heightened suspiciousness or a restriction in activity, social or a restriction in activity, social isolation, and loss of self-esteem.

2) Medical problems that mimic depression in the geriatric population:

   • increased sleep problems
   • decreased appetite
   • increased somatic concerns
   • slow and hesitate in movement
   • rigid in posture
   • tremulous

3) The blood volume falls with age, and there is a slight decline in hemoglobin concentration, more evident in women than men.

4) According to Eugen Bleuler, the four fundamental symptoms of psychoses:

   • Ambivalence
   • Disturbance of association
   • Disturbance of affect
   • Preference for fantasy over reality (autism)

5) Stages of the sexual response cycle:

   • Appetitive
   • Excitement

- Orgasm
- Resolution

6) There are decrements in dopaminergic functioning associated with age-related cell loss in the substantia nigra, with or without overt parkinsonian symptomatology.

7) Sleep disorders that are more common in the elderly:

   a) Nocturnal myoclonus
   b) Restless leg syndrome
   c) REM sleep behavior disturbance
   d) Sleep apnea
   e) Sundowning

8) The preoccupation of hypochondriasis may be with a specific organ or disease (e.g. cardiac disease), with bodily functions (e.g. peristalsis or heartbeat), or even with minor physical alterations (e.g. a small sore or an occasion cough). The fear becomes disabling and persists despite appropriate reassurance that no occasionally medical disease may be present.

9) Changing physiology in sexual relations with advancing age:

   - Men take longer to achieve an erection, and the erection is not as firm as it is in youth.
   - Intercourse is still pleasurable, although the ability to ejaculate decreases after age 60.
   - Following menopause, women experience atrophy of the vaginal mucosa, as well as a slower onset of lubrication.

10) Symptoms of depressed mood: dysphoria, tearfulness, and hopelessness. Symptoms of anxiety: psychic anxiety, palpations, jitteriness, or hyperventilation.

Chapter Nine: Psychiatric Treatments in the Elderly

Reference Notes

1) Questions required to answer:

   a) Does the patient have an ECT responsive illness?
   b) Does the patient have any medical problems that might require modifications of technique or increase the risks of the procedure?
   c) Has appropriate informed consent been obtained?

2) Common side effects of:

   - TCAs-sedation, orthostatic hypotension, and anticholinergic side effects such as constipation, urinary hesitancy, dry mouth, and visual blurring
   - SSRIs-Mild nausea, loose bowel movements, anxiety or hyperstimulation, headache sedation, and increased sweating.
   - MAOI's-Hypertensive crisis if tyramine restricted diet is not followed, orthostatic hypotension, insomnia or become irritable.

3) the most frequently used class of anxiolytic drugs are the benzodiazepines.

   a) Indications phobia, generalized anxiety, panic disorder, and obsessive-compulsive disorder
   b) Contra-indications lethal when combined with alcohol or other CNS depressants.

4) Patients with peptic ulcer disease or gastroesophageal reflux should receive their H2 blocker or metoclopramide with a

sip of water at least 2 hours before ECT. Then sodium citrate may be given immediately before treatment to neutralize any acid remaining in the stomach.

5) Special care required for psycopharmaceutical treatment:

Because renal and hepatic function show as a part of the normal aging process, medications for the geriatric population must be given in smaller doses than used for the general adult population.

6) Explain how ECT affects memory/ cognition in three ways:

   a) An acute postictal confusional state
   b) Anterograde memory dysfunction (AMD)
   c) Retrograde memory dysfunction (RMD)

7) Common extrapyramidal side effects that occur with antipsychotics: Falling, orthostatic side effects and sedating effects

8) Diagnoses in which ECT is considered ineffective:

   • Dementia and amnestic disorders
   • Substance-related disorders
   • Anxiety and somatiform disorders
   • Factitious disorders
   • Dissociative disorders
   • Sexual dysfunctions
   • Sleep disorders
   • Impulse disorders
   • Adjustment disorders
   • Personality disorders

9) Strategies that may be helpful if severe cognitive dysfunction develops:

- Switch from bilateral to unilateral electrode placement
- Decrease treatment frequency (from three times weekly to twice or once weekly)
- Decrease stimulus dose
- Review concurrent medications for contribution to cognitive dysfunction

10) Foods that will interact with an MAOI to produce a delirium:

- Aged chesses
- Beer, red wine, sherry, liqueurs
- Fermented sausage, beef or chicken liver, smoked or pickled fish, caviar
- Canned or overripe figs, whole bananas, banana peel fiber
- Fava or broad bean pods
- Yeast/Protein extracts

Chapter Ten: ECT in the Medically Ill Elderly

Reference Notes

1) The fact that ECT has clear anti-parkinsonian effects argues strongly for dopaminergic neurons of the nigrostriatal pathway, and the severe reduction of striatal dopamine and its metabolites, provided a rational basis for the development of dopamine replacement therapy in Parkinson's disease.

2) Cognitive function that presents when dementia coexists with depression:

    - Duration-days, weeks
    - Past history-affective illness
    - Neuro features-usually absent
    - Answers to questions-often I don't know
    - CT/ EEG-Usually normal
    - Response to antidepressant-Positive

3) Parameters used in the assessment of cardiac function before ECT:

    a) Conduction pattern
    b) Vascular supply
    c) Contractility
    d) Stress tolerance

4) Measures which are used in the assessment of congestive heart failure:

    a) An increased work load to which the heart cannot accommodate

b) A disorder of the myocardium so that it is unable to accommodate normal work loads

c) A restriction of ventricular filling so that an adequate stroke volume cannot be achieved.

5) Elderly patients have poor dentition and are at high risk for dental fracture. This is one of the commonest reasons for complaint or litigation in ECT patients.

- Some rubber bite blocks exert stress to the incisors during the stimulus and should be avoided.
- An alternative is a pair of rolled gauzes, one between each set of molars, which spare the incisors from mechanical stress

6) Meds and strategies for pulmonary management with ECT:

- Theophylline dosage should be decreased or discontinued before ECT because it lowers the seizure threshold and may be a cause of partial ictal activity or even status epilepticus after ECT
- If pulmonary management is required, then the patient should be observed for post-treatment seizure activity for several hours after treatment

7) Clinical features of Addison's disease:

- Hypotension
- Hyperkalemia
- Hyponatremia
- Low serum cortisol concentration

8) Depressions common at early stages of dementia and may frequently herald dementia onset. The emergence of

depression at any stage during dementia is usually associated with worsening cognitive performance and deteriorating function. Even when depressed mood is not evident, anxiety, sleep disturbance, or psychosis may be responsive to anti-depressants.

9) Clinical features of Parkinson's disease:

- Resting tremor rhythmically alternating contractions of a given muscle group
- Rigidity increased resistance to passive joint movement
- Akinesia disability or slowness in initiating movements, masked facies, decreased associated movements, e.g. arm-swinging while walking and stooped posture
- Loss of normal postural reflexes

10) Use of ECT in the treatment of epilepsy:

- The effects of ECT on seizure threshold have led to an understanding of the potent anti-convulsant properties of ECT
- For what seizure type would ECT be most effective partial or generalized?
- Would ECT effectively interrupt status epilepticus?
- What electrode placement and electrical dosing strategy would be optimal?
- What interval between maintenance treatments would be necessary to provide adequate protection against seizures?

Subject Index

Amnestic Syndrome

- Anterograde amnesia

- Psychogenic amnesia

- Retrograde amnesia

Anaphylactic shock

Anesthesia

Anesthetic agents

- Etomidate

- Ketamine

- Methohexital

- Propofol

- Thiopental

Aneurysms

Anorexia

Antianxiety drugs

Anticholinergic drugs

Anticonvulsant drugs

Biology of aging

Bradycardia

Brain biology

- Cerebral cortex

- Frontal lobes

- Occipital lobes

- Parietal lobes

- Temporal lobes

Brain Edema

- Cellular edema

- Cytotoxic edema

- Interstitial edema

- Vasogenic edema

Brain Location of ECT

- Left hemisphere

- Prefrontal cortex

- Right hemisphere

- Temporal lobe

Brief pulse square wave

C

Caffeine pretreatment

Carbamazepines

Carbohydrates

Cardiac arrhythmias

Cardiovascular diseases

Catactonic syndromes

Central nervous system diseases

Cerebrovascular diseases

Cerletti, Ugo

Cholinergic function

Chronic brain failure

Chronic bronchitis

Chronic obstructive pulmonary disease (COPD)

Clozapine

Colectomy

Congestive heart failure

Constipation

Convulsive Therapy

Coronary artery disease

Cortisol

Creutzfeldt-Jakob disease

Cuff technique

Cultural diversity

Cushing's syndrome

D

Delirium

Delirium tremens

Delusional disorders

Dementias

- Anterior dementias

- Axial dementias

- Cortical dementias

Geriatric Depression Scale

Geriatric drug metabolism

Glomerular Filtration Rate (GFR)

Golden Age of ECT

Goldman, Douglas

Grand Mal Seizure

Grave's Disease

H

Hallucinosis

Hartmann, Heinz

Headache

Hemingway, Ernest

Hemorrhage Sites

- Cerebellar hemorrhage

- Lobar hemorrhage

- Pontine Hemorrhage

- Putaminal Hemorrhage

- Thalamic Hemorrhage

Hepatic Synthesis

Hippocratic axiom

Histamine

Huntington's Chorea

Hypertension

Hyperventilate

Hypochondriasis

Hypoglycemic Shock

Hypomania

Hypotension

Hypothalamic-pituitary-adrenal axis

Hypothermia

I

Impedance

Informed consent

Insomnia

Insulin coma therapy

Muscle relaxant

Myocardinal infarction

N

National Alliance on Mental Illness

Nausea

Neurobiologic features

Neuroleptic Malignant Syndrome

Neuro-muscular blocking agents

Neurosyphilis

Neurotransmitter Therapy

Neurovegetative Functions

Niacin

Nocturnal myoclonus

Nonsteroidal anti-inflammatory drugs (NSAIDs)

Noradrenergic function

Norepinephrine

Normal Pressure Hydrocephalus

Nutrition

O

Obsessive-Compulsive Disorder

Orthostatic hypotension

Osteoporosis

Ottosson, JO

Outpatient ECT

Oxygen

Oxygenation

P

Paranoid Personality

Parkinson's Disease

Parisian Asylum Psychiatrists

Pascal, Constance

Pavlov, Ivan

Pellagra

Penicillin

Personality disorders

Petit mal Seizures

Pharmacokinetics

Pick's Disease

Pneumonia

Postictal care

Post-stroke depression

Post-Traumatic Stress Disorder (PTSD)

Pre-ECT Evaluation

Prodromal Phase

Progressive Strokes

Propofol

Proteins

Pseudodementias

Psychoanalysis

Psychoneurses

Psychotherapy

Psychotic depression

Pulmonary Diseases

R

Reserpine

Residual Phase

Restless Leg Syndrome

Reversible Ischemic Neurologic Deficit

Rosenberg, Leon

S

Sackeim, Harold

Safe environment

Saffron extract

Sakel, Manfred

Schizoid Personality

Schizophrenia

- Negative symptoms

- Positive symptoms

Schuster, Julius

Seizure threshold

Selective Serotonin Reuptake Inhibitor (SSRI)

Serotonin

Sexual dysfunction

Sexual Response Phase

Shock docs

Shock therapy

Side effects of ECT

Sine wave

Sinusoidal waveforms

Sleep apnea

Sleep disturbances

Sleep hygiene

Small airways disease

Somatotherapies

Steck, Hans

Stimulus waveform

Stroke-in-evaluation

Thyrotoxicosis

Tonic-clonic muscle contractions

Transient Ischemic Attacks (TIA)

Tranquilizers

Trytophan

Turmeric

Tyramine

Tyrosine

U

U.S. Public Health Service Survey

V

Valproate

Vasconcellos, John

Vascular dementia

Vascular Depression Hypothesis

Ventricular Arrythmia

Vital Signs

W

Wagner-Jauregg, Julius

Weiner, Richard

World War I

World War II

Bibliography

Abraham G, Milev R, Delva N, et al. Clinical Outcome and Memory Function with Maintenance Electroconvulsive Therapy: A Retrospective Study. The Journal of ECT, 22: 43-45, 2006.

Abrams R. Special issue on the high-risk patient. Convulsive Therapy 5 (entire issue), 1989.

Abrams R. Daily administration of unilateral ECT. American Journal of Psychiatry 124:384-386, 1967.

Abrams R and Swartz CM. ECT and prolactin release: relation to treatment response in melancholia. Convulsive Therapy 1: 38-42, 1985.

Abrams R. Electroconvulsive Therapy. New York, Oxford University Press, 1988.

Abrams R, Taylor MA, Faber R, et al. Bilateral versus unilateral electroconvulsive therapy: efficacy in melancholia. American Journal of Psychiatry 140: 463-465, 1983.

Abrams R, Swartz CM, Vedak C. Antidepressant effects of high-dose right unilateral electroconvulsive therapy. Archives General Psychiatry 48: 746-748, 1991.

Abrams R. Efficacy of electroconvulsive therapy. In: Electroconvulsive Therapy, 4th ed. New York: Oxford University Press, 17-42, 2002.

Abrams R (ed). Special Issue on the High-Risk Patient. Convulsive Therapy 5 (entire Issue), 1989.

Abrams R. ECT for Parkinson's disease. American Journal of Psychiatry 146: 1391-1393, 1989.

Abrams R. Electroconvulsive Therapy 2nd Edition, New York, Oxford University Press, 1992.

Abrams R. Electroconvulsive Therapy. Oxford University Press, 2002.

Acevedo AG, Smith JK. Adverse-reaction to use of caffeine in ECT. American Journal of Psychiatry. 145: 529-30, 1988.

Addersley DJ, Hamilton M. Use of succinylcholine in ECT. British Medical Journal. 1: 195-195, 1953.

Addonizio G, Alexopoulos GS. Affective disorders in the elderly. International Journal of Psychiatry 8: 41, 1993.

Aden, Gary C. The International Psychiatric Association for the Advancement of Electrotherapy: A Brief History. American Journal of Social Psychiatry 4 (Fall 1984).

Alexopoulos GS, Meyer BS, Young RC, et al. Vascular depression hypothesis. Archives of General Psychiatry 54: 915-922, 1997.

Alexopoulos GS, Meyer BS, Young RC, et al. Clinically defined vascular depression. American Journal of Psychiatry 154: 562-565, 1997.

Alexopoulos GS. Depression in the elderly. Lancet 365: 1961-1970, 2005.

Alexopoulus GS, Young RC, Abrams RC. ECT in the high risk geriatric population. Convulsive Therapy 5: 75-87, 1989.

Alexopoulos GS, Shamoian CJ, Lucas J, Weiser N, Berger H. Medical problems of geriatric psychiatric patients and younger controls during electroconvulsive therapy. Journal of America Geriatric Society 32: 651-4, 1984.

Alger I. History of modern psychiatry, and modern application of electroconvulsive treatment. Hospital and Community Psychiatry. 42: 355-356, 1991.

American Psychiatric Association. The Practice of Electroconvulsive Therapy: Recommendations for treatment, training, and privileging. A Task Force Report of the American Psychiatric Association. Washington, DC, American Psychiatric Association, 1990.

American Psychiatric Association. Diagnostic and Statistical Manual of Mental Disorders, Text Revision, 4th ed, American Psychiatric Association, 2000.

American Psychiatric Association: The Practice of Electroconvulsive Therapy: Recommendations for Treatment, Training, and Privileging. A Task Force Report of the American Psychiatric Association. Washington, DC, American Psychiatric Association, 1990.

American Psychiatric Association. Diagnostic and Statistical Manual of Mental Disorders, 5th ed. Washington, DC: American Psychiatric Publishing. 197-202, 2013.

American Psychiatric Association. (APA). Electroconvulsive Therapy: Fact Sheet, October, 1997.

American Psychiatric Association, Task Force on Electroconvulsive Therapy: The Practice of Electroconvulsive Therapy: Recommendations for Treatment, Training, and Privileging. Washington, DC, 1990.

Andersen K, Balldin J, Gottfries CG, et al. A double-blind evaluation of electroconvulsive therapy in Parkinson's Disease with "on-off" phenomena. Acta Nuerol Scand 76: 191-199, 1987.

Andrade C and Kurinji S. Continuation and Maintenance ECT: A Review of Recent Research. The Journal of ECT, 18 (3): 149-158, 2002.

Asnis G. Parkinson's disease, depression, and ECT: a review and case study. American Journal Psychiatry 134: 191-195, 1977.

Association for Convulsive Therapy: Task Force Report on Ambulatory Electroconvulsive Therapy. Convulsive Therapy 12: 42-55, 1996.

Astrom M, Adolfsson R, Asplund K. Major depression in stroke patients. A 3 year longitudinal study. Stroke 24: 976-982, 1993.

Aziz M, Mehringer AM, Mozurkewich E, et al. Cost-utility of 2 maintenance treatments for older adults with depression who responded to a course of electroconvulsive therapy: results from a decision analytic model. Canada Journal of Psychiatry 50: 389-397, 2005.

Bajbouj M, Lang UE, Niehaus L, et al. Effects of right unilateral electroconvulsive therapy on motor cortical excitability in depressive patients. Journal of Psychiatry Research. 40: 322-327, 2006

Barclay TH, Barclay RD. A clinical trial of cranial electrotherapy trial of cranial electrotherapy stimulation for anxiety and comorbid depression. Journal of Affective Disorders. 164: 171-77, 2014.

Barton JL. ECT in depression: The evidence of controlled studies. Biol Psychiatry 12: 687-95, 1977.

Baxter, Lewis R. Roy-Byrne P. Liston EH. and Fairbanks L. The Experience of Electroconvulsive Therapy in the 1980's: A Propective Study of the Knowledge, Opinions, and Experience of California Electroconvulsive Therapy. Patients in Berkely Years. Convulsive Therapy 2, no 3 (1986).

Beale MD, Bernstein JH, Kellner CH. Maintenance ECT for geriatric depression: a one year follow-up. Clinical Gerontologist 16: 86-90, 1996.

Beale MD, Kellner CH. Electroconvulsive therapy and drug interactions. Psychiatric Clinic North America 3: 119-131, 1996.

Belvederi Murri M, Respino M, Masotti M, et al. Vitamin D and psychosis: mini meta-analysis. Schizophrenia Research. 150(1): 235-39, 2013.

Benbow S. The use of electroconvulsive therapy in old age psychiatry. International Journal of Geriatric Psychiatry 2: 25-30, 1987.

Benbow S. ECT for depression in dementia (letter). British Journal of Psychiatry 152: 859, 1988.

Benbow SM. The use of electroconvulsive therapy in old age psychiatry. International Journal of Geriatric Psychiatry 2: 25030, 1987.

Benbow SM. ECT for depression in dementia. British Journal of Psychiatry 152: 85-9, 1987.

Beresford HR. Legal Issues relating to electroconvulsive therapy. Archives of General Psychiatry, 25: 100-102, 1971.

Bidder TG, Strain JJ, and Brunschwig L. Bilateral and Unilateral ECT: Follow-up Study and Critique. American Journal of Psychiatry. 127, no 6 (1970).

Bielski V. Electroshock's Quiet Comeback. San Francisco Bay Guardian, April 18, 1990.

Blachly PH. New Development in electroconvulsive therapy. Disorders Nervous System 37: 356-358, 1976.

Blumenthal JA, Babyak MA, Moore KA, et al. Effects of exercise training on older patients with major depression. Archives of Internal Medicine. 159 (19): 2349-56, 1999.

Boccio R, Fink M. A comparison of etomidate and methohexital anesthesia for electroconvulsive therapy. Ann Clinical Psychiatry 1:39-42, 1989.

Boey WK, Lai FO. Comparison of propofol and thiopentone as anaesthetic agents for electroconvulsive therapy. Anaesthesia 45: 623-628, 1990.

Bolwig TG. How does electroconvulsive therapy work? Theories on its mechanism. Canada Journal of Psychiatry 56: 13-18, 2011.

Bonds C, Frye M, Coudreaut MF, et al. Cost reduction in refractory bipolar disorder. Journal of ECT. 14: 36-41, 1998.

Bostwick JM, and Pankratz VS. Affective disorders and suicide risk. A re-examination. American Journal of Psychiatry, 157: 1925-1932, 2000.

Bouckoms AJ, Welch CA, Drop LJ, et al. Atropine in electroconvulsive therapy. Convulsive Therapy 5: 48-55, 1989.

Boylan LS, Haskett RF, Mulsant BH, et al. Determinants of seizure threshold in ECT: benzodiazepine use, anesthetic dosage, and other factors. Journal of ECT 16: 3-18, 2000.

Breakey WR and Dunn G. Racial disparity in the use of ECT for affective disorders. American Jouranl of Psychiatry (in Press).

Bross MH, Tatum NO. Delirium in the elderly patient. American Family Physician. 50: 1325-1332, 1994.

Brown GL and Wilson WP. Parkinsonism and depression. South Medical Journal 65: 540-545, 1972.

Burke WJ, Rubin EH, Zorumski CF, Wetzel RD. The safety of ECT in geriatric psychiatry. Journal of American Geriatric Society. 35: 516-21, 1987.

Burke WJ, Rutherford JL, Zorumski CF, Reich T. Electroconvulsive therapy and the elderly. Compr Psychiatry 26: 480-6, 1985.

Calev A, Drexler H, Tubi N, et al. Atropine and cognitive performance after electroconvulsive therapy. Convulsive Therapy 7: 92-98, 1991.

Cannicott SM, Waggoner RW. Unilateral and bilateral electroconvulsive therapy. Archive General Psychaitry. 16: 229-32, 1967.

Casey DA, Davis MH. Electroconvulsive Therapy in the very old. General Hospital Psychiatry 18 (6); 436-439, 1996.

Cerletti U. Electroshock Therapy. Journal of Clinical Experiments 15. No 3. Sept, 1954.tria Argentina 2: 292-296, 1956.

Chang BH, Sommers E. Acupuncture and relaxation response for craving and anxiety reduction among military veterans in recovery from substance use disorder. The American Journal of Addictions 23 (2): 129-36, 2014.

Clark CO, Alexopoulus GS, Kaplan J. Prolactin release and clinical response to electroconvulsive therapy in depressed geriatric inpatients: A preliminary report. Convulsive Therapy. 11: 24-31, 1995.

Clark L, Chamberlain SR, Sahakian BJ. Neurocogntive mechanisms in depression: implications for treatment. Annual Review of Neuroscience 32: 57-74, 2009.

Clayton PJ. Suicide. Psychiatry Clinic North America 8: 203-214, 1985.

Clinical Trial of the Treatment of Depressive Illness: Report to the Medical Research Council by the Its Clinical Psychiatry Committee. British Medical Journal 1, 1965.

Clyma EA. Unilateral electroconvulsive therapy: how to determine which hemisphere is dominant. British Journal of Psychiatry 126: 372-379, 1975

Coffey CE, ed. The Clinical Science of Electroconvulsive Therapy. Washington, DC: American Psychiatric Press, 1993.

Coffey CE. The Clinical Science of Electroconvulsive Therpay. American Psychiatric Press, Inc. 1993.

Coffey CE, Figiel GS, Weiner RD, et al. Caffeine augmentation of electroconvulsive therapy. American Journal of Psychiatry 147: 579-585, 1990.

Coffey CE and Weiner RD. Electroconvulsive Therapy: An update. Hospital and Community Psychiatry. 41, no 5. May, 1990.

Coffey CE, Figiel GS, Weiner RD. Saunders WB. Caffeine augmentation of ECT. American Journal of Psychiatry. 147:579-85, 1990.

Coffey CE, Figiel GS, Weiner RD, et al. Caffeine augmentation of ECT. American Journal of Psychiatry 147: 579-585, 1990.

Colantonio A, Kasi SV, Ostfeld AM, et al. Psychosocial predictors of stroke outcomes in an elderly population. Journal of Gerontol 48: S261-S268, 1993.

Cronin D, Bodley P, Potts L, et al. Unilateral and bilateral ECT: a study of memory disturbance and relief from depression. Journal Neurol Neurosurg Psychiatry. 33: 705-711, 1970.

Coffey CE, Weiner RD, Hinkle PE, Cress M, Daughtry G, Wilson WH. Augmentation of ECT seizures with caffeine. Biol Psychiatry. 22: 637-49, 1987.

Coffey CE, Weiner RD, Hinkle PE, et al. Augmentation of ECT seizures with caffeine. Biol Psychiatry 22: 637-649, 1987.

Coffey CE, Figiel GS, Weiner RD, et al. Caffeine augmentation of electroconvulsive therapy. American Journal of Psychiatry 147:579-585, 1990.

Coffey CE, Figiel GS, Weiner RD, et al. Caffeine augmentation of ECT. American Journal of Psychiatry 147: 579-585, 1990.

Cohen D. Electroconvulsive Treatment, Neurology and Psychiatry. Ethical Human Science and Service. 3, no.2. 2001.

Creutzfeldt O, Ojemann G. Neuronal activity in the human lateral temporal lobe III. Activity changes during music. Experimental Brain Research. 77(3): 490-98, 1989.

Culver CM, Ferrell RB and Green RM. ECT and special problems of informed consent. The American Journal of Psychiatry. 137, 586-591, 1980.

Daniel WF, Crovitz HF. Acute memory impairment following electroconvulsive therapy, 2: effect of electrode placement. Acta Psychiatry Scand 67: 57-68, 1983.

Davis J, Janicak P, Sakkas P, et al. Electroconvulsive therapy in the treatment of the neuroleptic malignant syndrome. Convulsive Therapy 7: 111-120, 1991

Davis PH et al. Risk factors for ischemic stroke: a propesctive study in Rochester, Minnesota. Ann Neurol 22: 319, 1982.

D'Elia G, Raotma H. Is Unilateral ECT less effective than bilateral ECT? British Journal of Psychiatry 126: 83-89, 1975.

Devanand DP, Fitzsimons L, Prudic J, and Sackeim HA. Subjective Side Effects During Electroconvulsive Therapy. Convulsive Therapy. 11, no.4. 1995.

Delva NJ, Brunet D, Hawken ER, et al. Electrical dose and seizure threshold: relations to clinical outcome and cognitive effects in bifrontal, bitemporal, and right unilateral ECT. Journal of ECT 16: 361-369, 2000.

De Quardo JR, Tandon R. ECT in post-stroke major depression. Convulsive Therapy 4: 221-224, 1988.

Donahue AB. Electroconvulsive therapy and memory loss: a personal journey. Journal of ECT 16: 133-143, 2000.

Donahue AB. A Basic Layperson's Guide to Decision Making About ECT, Including Key Questions to Ask Your Doctor, undated.

Drop Welch CA. Anesthesia for electroconvulsive therapy in patients with major cardiovascular risk factors. Convulsive Therapy 5: 88-101, 1989.

Dubovsky S. Using electroconvulsive therapy for patients with neurological disease. Hospital Community Psychiatry. 37: 819-824, 1986.

Dukakis K. and Tye L. Shock: The Healing Power of Electroconvulsive Therapy. The Penguin Group, 2006.

Dukakis K, Tye L. Shock: the healing power of electroconvulsive therapy. New York: Avery, 2006.

Duncan AJ, Ungvari GS, Russell RJ, et al. Maintenance ECT in very old age: case report. Annals of Clinical Psychiatry 2: 139-144, 1990.

Duncan AJ, Ungvari GS, Russell RJ, et al. Maintenance ECT in very old age: case report. Annals of Clinical Psychiatry 2:139-144, 1990.

Durr AL and Golden RN. Cognitive Effects of Electroconvulsive Therapy: A Clinical Review for Nurses. Convulsive Therapy II, no. 3. 1995.

Durr AL and Golden RN. Cognitive Effects of Electroconvulsive Therapy: A Clinical Review for Nurses. Conclusive Therapy II. No.3. 1995.

Egbert LD, Wolfe S. Evaluation of Methohexital for premedication in electroshock therapy. Anesth Analg 39: 416-419, 1960.

Ellgring H, Seiler S, Perleth B, et al. Psychosocial aspects of Parkinson's disease. Neurology 43: S41-S44, 1993.

Endler NS. The origins of electroconvulsive therapy (ECT). Convulsive Therapy. 4: 5-23.

Engel JE, Jr. Seizures and epilepsy. Philadelphia: FA Davis, 1989.

Eranti SV and McLoughlin DM. Electroconvulsive Therapy—State of the Art. British Journal of Psychiatry 182, 2003.

Eranti SV and McLoughlin DM. Electroconvulsive Therapy—State of the Art. British Journal of Psychiatry 182. 2003.

Eranti SV, Mogg AJ, Pluck GC, et al. Methohexitone, propofol and etomidate in electroconvulsive therapy for depression: a naturalistic comparison study. Journal Affective Disorder 113: 165-171, 2009.

Evans LK. Sundown syndrome in institutionalized elderly. Journal of American Geriatric Society. 35: 101-108, 1987.

Faber R and Trimble M, Electroconvulsive therapy in Parkinson's Disease and other movement disorders. Movement Disorders. 6: 293-303, 1991.

Faber R, Trimble M. Electroconvulsive therapy in Parkinson's disease and other movement disorders. Movement Disorders 6: 293-303, 1991.

Fakhri O, Fadhli A, Rawi R. Effect of elctroconvulsive therapy on diabetes mellitus. Lancet 2: 775-777, 1980.

Farah A and Mc Call WV. Electroconvulsive Therapy Stimulus Dosing: A survey of Contemporary Practices. Convulsive Therapy 9, no.2. (1993).

Farrell KR and Ganzini L. Misdiagnosing delirium as depression in medically ill elderly patients. Archive Internal Meidcine. 155: 2459-2464, 1995.

Fawcett J, Clark DC, Busch KA. Assessing and treating the patient at risk for suicide. Psychiatry Ann. 23: 244-255, 1993.

Feinberg M, Gillin JC, Carrol BJ, et al. EEG studies of sleep in the diagnosis of depression. Biological Psychiatry 305-316, 1982.

Figiel GS, Stoydemire A. The use of ECT for elderly patients with cardiac disease. Psychiatric Times, 13-7. December, 1994.

Finestone DH, Weiner RD. Effects of ECT on diabetes mellitus. Acta Psychiatry Scand. 70: 321-326, 1984.

Fink M and Johnson L. Monitoring the Duration of Electroconvulsive Therapy Seizures. Archives of General Psychiatry 39, no.10. (1982).

Fink M. Electroconvulsive Therapy: A Guide for Professionals and Their Patients. Oxford University Press, 2009.

Fink M. Electroshock: Restoring the Mind, Oxford University Press, 1999.

Fink M. Reversible and Irreversible dementia. Convulsive Therapy. 5: 123-125, 1989.

Fleminger JJ, deHorne DJ, Nair NPV, et al. Differential effect of Unilateral and Bilateral ECT. American Journal of Psychiatry 127: 430-436, 1970.

Fochtmann L. A mechanism for the efficacy of ECT in Parkinson's disease. Convulsive Therapy. 4: 321-327, 1988.

Fochtmann L. A mechanism for the efficacy of ECT in Parkinson's disease. Convulsive Therapy. 4: 321-327, 1988.

Folk JW Kellner CH, Beale MD, et al. Anesthesia for electroconvulsive therapy: a review. Journal of ECT 16: 157-170, 2000.

Folstein MF and Ross C. Cognitive Impairment in the elderly. In textbook of Internal Medicine, 2nd ed. Kelley Wm, ed. Philadelphia: JB Lippincott, 2408-2410, 1992.

Fox HA. Continuation and Maineneance ECT. Jouran of Practical Psychiatry and Behavioral Health, 1996.

Fox HA, Rosen A. Campbell RJ. Are brief pulse and sine wave ECT equally efficient? Journal of Clinical Psychiatry 50: 432-435, 1989.

Frankel FH. Current Perspectives on ECT: Discussion. American Journal of Psychaitry. 134, no.9 (1977).

Francis J, Kapor WN. Delirium in hospitalized elderly. Journal of General Internal Medicine 5: 65, 1990.

Francis J, Kapoor WN. Delirium in hospitalized elderly. Journal of Intern Medicine 5:65, 1990.

Fraser M. ECT: A Clinical Guide. New York: John Wiley= Sons, 1982.

Fraser RM, Glass IB. Unilateral and bilateral ECT in elderly patients. A comparative study. Acta Psychiatry Scand. 62: 13-31, 1980.

French J. The long-term therapeutic management of epilepsy. Ann Intern Med 120: 411, 1994.

Gaines GY, Rees I. Electroconvulsive therapy in the medically ill elderly. Convulsive Therapy 5: 8-16, 1989.

Gaines GY, Rees I. Electroconvulsive therapy and anesthetic considerations. Anesthesia Analg 65: 1345-1356, 1986.

Garcia-Ptacek S, Faxen Irving G, Cermakova P, et al. Body mass index in dementia. European Journal of Clinical Nutrition. 68 (11): 1204-9, 2014.

Gass JP. The Knowledge and Attitudes of Mental Health Nurses to Electroconvulsive Therapy. Journal of Advanced Nursing, 27, no. 1. 1998.

Geddes JR. Efficacy and safety of electroconvulsive therapy in depressive disorders: A systematic review and meta-analysis. The Lancet, 361: 700-808, 2003.

Gilbert DT. Shock therapy and informed consent. Illinois Bar Jouranl. January: 272-87, 1981.

Glass RM. Electroconvulsive Therapy: Time to Bring It Out of the Shadows. Journal of American Medical Association, 285, no.10. 2001.

Goldberg R. Geriatric consultation/ Liaison psychiatry. Adv Psychosom Med 19: 138, 1989.

Goldman D. Brief stimulus electric shock therapy. Journal of Nerve Mental Disorder 110: 36-45, 1949

Gorelick PB. Etiology and management of acute stroke. Compr Ther 15: 60-65, 1989.

Gosek E, Weller R. Improvement of tardive dyskinesia associated with electroconvulsive therapy. Journal of Nerve Movement Disorders 176: 120-122, 1988.

Greenberg MK, Barsan WG, Starkman S. Neuroimaging in the emergency patient presenting with seizure. Neurology 47: 26-32, 1996.

Greenberg RM and Kellner CH. Electroconvulsive Therapy: A Selected Review. American Journal of Geriatric Psychiatry 13, no.4. 2005.

Group for the Advancement of Psychiatry. Revised Electro-Shock Therapy Report. Report No. 15. New York, 1947.

Guttmacher LB, Greenland P. Effects of electroconvulsive therapy on the electrocardiogram in geriatric patients with stable cardiovascular diseases. Convulsive Therapy 6: 5-12, 1990.

Gu Y, Nieves JW, Stern Y, et al. Food combination and Alzheimer disease risk: a protective diet. Archives of Neurology 67 (6): 699-706, 2010.

Hamilton M. A rating scale for depression. Journal Neurol Neurosurg Psychiatry 23: 56-62, 1960.

Harms E. The Origin and Early History of Electrotherapy and Electroshock. American journal of Psychiatry III, no. 12. 1955.

Hawton K. Assessment of suicide risk. British Journal of Psychiatry. 150:145-153. 1987.

Hay DP. Electroconvulsive therapy in the medically ill elderly. Convulsive Therapy 5: 8-16, 1989.

Heinbecker P. The pathogenesis of Cushing's disease. Medicine 23: 225, 1944.

Herman RC, Dorwart RA, Hoover CW, and Brody J. Variation in ECT use in the United States. American Journal of Psychiatry 152. No.6. 1995.

Herman RC, Ettner SL, Dorwart RA, Hoover CW, and Yeung E. Characteristics of Psychiatrists who perform ECT. American Journal of Psychiatry 155, no.7. 1998.

Himwich HE. Electroshock: A Round Table Discussion. American Journal of Psychiatry 100. 1943.

Hinkle PE, Coffey CE, Weiner RD, et al. Use of caffeine to lengthen seizures in ECT. American Journal of Psychiatry 144: 1143-1148, 1987.

Iliff J. One more reason to get a good night's sleep. In TED, editior, 2014.

illikan CH, Mc Dowell FH. Treatment of progressing stroke. Stroke 12: 397, 1981.

Irish M, Hodges JR, Piquet O. Right anterior temporal lobe dysfunction underlies theory of mind impairments in semantic dementia. Brain: A Journal of Neurology, 1241-53, 2014.

Jacobson SA. Delirium in the elderly. Psychiatric Clinic North America. 20: 91-110, 1997.

Jaffe R, Dubin W, Shoyer B, et al. Outpatient electroconvulsive therapy: efficacy and safety. Convulsive Therpay 6: 231-238, 1990.

Jackson J. Electroconvulsive Therapy: Problems and Prejudices. Convulsive Therapy II, no.3 1995.

Jamison KR. An Unquiet Mind: A Memoir of Moods and Madness. New York: Vintage Books, 1995.

Janouschek H, Nicki-Jockschat T, Haeck M, et al. Comparison of methohexital and etomidate as anesthetic agents for electroconvulsive therapy in affective and psychotic disorders. Journal of Psychiatry Research 47: 686-693, 2013.

Kales H. Raz J, Tandon R, et al. Relationship of seizure duration to antidepressant efficacy in electroconvulsive therapy. Psychol Medicine 27: 1373-80, 1997.

Kalinowky LB. History of convulsive therapy. Ann NY Acad Science 462:1-4, 1986.

Kamil R, Joffe RT. Neuroendocrine testing in electroconvulsive therapy. Psychiatry Clinic North America 14: 887-903, 1991.

Karliner W. Maintenance ECT. Journal of Psychiatric Treatment and Evaluation 2: 313-314, 1980.

Kellner CH. Pritchett JT, Beale MD, Coffey CE. Handbook of ECT. American Psychiatric Press, Inc. 1997.

Kellner CH. Electroconvulsive therapy. Psychiatric Clinic North American 14 (entire issue), 1991.

Kellner CH. (ed). ECT and Drugs: Concurrent Administration. Convulsive Therapy 9: 237-240, 1993.

Kellner CH. ECT at a mid-Decade: Two Steps Forward. One Step Back. Convulsive Therapy II, no.1. 1995.

Kellner CH, Greenberg RM, Murrough JW, et al. ECT in treatment –resistant depression. American Journal of Psychiatry. 169: 1238-1244, 2012.

Kellner CH, Fink M, Knapp R, et al. Relief of expressed suicidal intent by ECT: a consortium for research in ECT study. American Journal of Psychiatry. 162: 977-982, 2005.

Kesey K. One Flew over the Cuckoo's Nest. New York: Viking Press, 1962.

Kessler U, Schoeyen HK, Andreassen OA, et al. The effect of electroconvulsive therapy on neurocognitive function in treatment-resistant bipolar disorder depression, Journal Clinical of Psychiatry 75: e 1306-e1313, 2014.

Klainin-Yobas P, Oo WN, Suzanne Yew PY, et al. Effects of relaxation interventions on depression and anxiety among older adults: a systematic review. Aging and Mental Health. 1-3, 2015.

King BH, Liston EH, Proposals for the mechanism of action of electroconvulsive therapy: a synthesis. Biol Psychiatry. 27: 76-94, 1990.

Kivler CA. Will I ever be the same again? Transforming the Face of ECT (Shock Therapy) Three Gem publishing/ Kivler Communications, 2010.

Koenig HG, Breitner JC. Use of antidepressants in medically ill older patients. Psychosomatics 31: 22, 1990.

Kramer BA. Maintenance electroconvulsive therapy in clinical practice. Convulsive Therapy 6: 279-286, 1990.

Kramer BA. Outpatient electroconvulsive therapy: a cost saving alternative. Hospital Community Psychiatry 41: 361-363, 1990.

Kroessler D and Fogel BS. Electroconvulsive Therapy for Major Depression In the Oldest Old: Effects of Medical Comorbidity on Post-Treatment Survival. American Journal of Geriatric Psychiatry 1, no.1.1993.

Knos GB, Sung YF. ECT Anesthesia strategies in the high risk medical patient. In: Psychiatric Care of the Medical Patient, Stoudemire A, Fogel BS, eds. New York: Oxford University Press, 1993.

Landy DA. Combined use of Clozapine and Electroconvulsive therapy, 7: 218-221, 1991.

Lauterbach E, Moore N. Parkinsonism-dystonia syndrome and ECT. American Journal Psychiatry. 147: 1249-1250, 1990.

Lawson JS, Inglis J, Delva NJ, et al. Electrode placement in ECT: cognitive effects. Psycho Med 20: 335-344, 1990.

Lebensohn ZM. The History of Electroconvulsive Therapy in the United States and Its Place in American Psychiatry: A Personal Memoir. Comprehensive Psychiatry 40, no. 3, 1999.

Levy L, Savit J, Hodes M. Parkinsonism: improvement by electroconvulsive therapy. Archives of Phys Med Rehabil. 64: 432-433, 1983.

Liggan DY, Kay J. Depression in the Elderly: Diagnosis and Treatment. Hospital Physician. Psychiatry Board Review Manual. Turner White Communications, Inc. 1999.

Lipowski ZJ. Delirium in the elderly patient. New England Journal of Medicine. 320: 578-582, 1989.

Lisanby SH and Morales OG. Invited Review of Electroconvulsive Therapy by Richard Abrams. Psychological Medicine 33, 2003.

Lisanby SH and Morales OG. Invited Review of Electroconvulsive Therapy by Richard Abrams. Psychological Medicine 33, 2003.

Lisanby S. Electroconvulsive therapy for depression. New England Journal of Medicine. 357: 1939-1945, 2007.

Loo H, Galinowski A, DeCarvalho W, Bourdel MC, Poirier MF. Use of maintenance ECT for elderly depressed patients. American Journal Psychiatry 148: 810, 1991.

Luhdorf K, Jensen LK, Plesner AM. Epilepsy in the Elderly: etiology of seizures in elderly. Epilepsia 27: 458, 1986.

MacEwan T. An audit of seizure duration in elctorconvulsive therapy. Psychiatric Bulletin 26: 337-339, 2002.

Maneksha FR. Hypertension and tachycardia during electroconvulsive therapy: to treat or not to treat? Convulsive Therapy 7: 28-35, 1991.

Maletzky BM. Seizure duration and clinical effect in electroconvulsive therapy. Compr Psychiatry 19: 541-550, 1978.

Malsch E, Ho L, Booth MJ, and Allen E. Survey of Anesthetic Coverage of Electroconvulsive Therapy in the State of Pennsylvania. Convulsive Therapy 7, No. 4. 1991.

Malitz S, Sackeim HA, Decina P. ECT in the treatment of major affective disorders: clinical and basic research issues. Psychiatric Journal Univeraity of Ottawa 7: 126-134, 1982.

Manly T and Swartz CM. Asymmetric bilateral right frontotemporal left frontal stimulus electrode placement: comparisons with bifrontotemporal and unilateral placements. Convulsion Therapy 10(4): 267-270, 1994.

Manly T, Oakley SP Jr, Bloch RM. Electroconvulsive therapy in old-old age patients. American Journal of Geriatric Psychiatry 8(3): 232-236, 2000.

Maxwell RD. Electrical factors in electroconvulsive therapy. Acta Psychiatry Scand 44: 436-448, 1968.

McAllister DA, Perri MG, Jordan MC, et al. Effects of ECT given two vs. three times weekly. Psychiatry Research 21: 63-69, 1987.

Mc Donald WM, Phillips VL, Figiel GS, et al. Cost-effective maintenance treatment of resistant geriatric depression. Psychiatry Ann 28: 47-52, 1998.

McCall WV, Reid S, Rosenquist P, et al. A reappraisal of the role of caffeine in ECT. American Journal of Psychiatry 150: 1543-1545, 1993.

McLean Hospital Archives. Electric Shock Treatment Procedure. Undated. Belmont, Massachussets.

McLean Hospital Archives. General Preparatory Requirements and Consideration for Electric Shock Therapy at the Mclean Hospital. Undated.

Miller AL, Faber RA, Hatch JP, et al. Factors affecting amnesia, seizure duration, and efficacy in ECT. American Journal of Psychiatry. 142: 692-696, 1985.

Millikan CH, McDowell FH. Treatment of Progressing Stroke. Stroke. 12:397, 1981.

Mitchell P, Smythe G, Torda T. Effect of the anesthetic agent propofol on hormonal responses to ECT. Biol of Psychiatry 28: 315-324, 1990.

Mitchell P, Torda T, Hickie I, et al. Propofol as an anesthetic agent for ECT: effect on outcome and length of course. Australia New Zealand Journal of Psychiatry 25: 255-261, 1991.

Monroe RR. Maintenance electroconvulsive therapy. Psychiatry Clin North America. 14: 947-960, 1991.

Monroe RR. Maintenance electroconvulsive therapy. Psychiatric Clinic North American 14: 947-960, 1991.

Morris V. How to care for Aging Parents. Workman Publishing: New York, 2004.

Moscicki EK. Epidemiology of suicidal behavior. Suicide Life Threat Behavior. 25: 22-35, 1995.

Moscicki EK. Gender differences in completed and attempted suicides. Ann Epidemiol 4: 152-158, 1994

Murray GB, Shea V, Conn DK. Electroconvulsive therapy for post-stroke depression. Journal of Clinical Psychiatry 47: 258-260, 1986.

National Institute of Health. Electroconvulsive Therapy: National Institutes of Health Consensus Development Conference Statements. 5 (11): 1-23. 1985.

National Institutes of Health Consensus Development Panel on Depression in Late Life. Diagnosis and Treatment of Depression in Late Life. Journal of the American Medical Association 268, no 8. 1992.

Niedermeyer E. The Epilepsies. Diagnosis and Management. Baltimore, Urban and Schwarzenberg, 1990.

Nelson JP, Rosenberg DR. ECT treatment of demented elderly patients with major depression. Convulsive Therapy 7: 157-165, 1991.

Nelson JP, Benjamin L. Efficacy and safety of combined ECT and tricyclic antidepressant drugs in the treatment of depressed drugs in the treatment of depressed geriatric patients. Convulsive Therapy 5: 321-329, 1989.

Nelson JP, Rosenberg DR. ECT treatment of demented elderly patients with major depression: a retrospective study of efficacy and safety. Convulsive Therapy 7: 157-165, 1991.

Nettelbladt P. Factors influencing number of treatments and seizure duration in ECT: drug treatment, social class. Convulsive Therapy 4: 160-168, 1988.

Nobler MS, Sackeim HA, Solomou M, Luber B, et al. EEG manifestations during ECT: effects of electrode placement and stimulus intensity. Biol Psychiatry 34: 321-340, 1993.

Ottosson JO and Fink M. Ethics in Electroconvulsive Therapy. Brunner-Routedge, 2004.

Pan W, Kastin AJ. Can sleep apnea cause Alzheimer's disease? Neuroscience and Biobehavioral Reviews. 47C: 656-69, 2014.

Patel M, Patel S, Hardy DW, et al. Should electroconvulsive therapy be an early consideration for suicidal patients? Journal of ECT, 22: 113-115, 2006.

Petrides G, Tobias KG, Kellner CH, et al. Continuation and maintenance electroconvulsive therapy for mood disorders: a review of the literature. Neuropsychobiology, 64: 129-140, 2011.

Petrides G. Continuation ECT: A review. Psychiatric Annals. 28: 517-523, 1998.

Pettinati HM, Bonner KM. Cognitive functioning in depressed geriatric patients with history of ECT. American Journal of Psychiatry 141: 49-52, 1984.

Philbert RA, Richards L, Lynch CF, and Winokur G. Effect of ECT on Mortality and Clinical Outcome in Geriatric Unipolar Depression. Journal of Clinical Psychiatry 56, no. 9. 1995.

Philot M, Treloar A, Gormley, and Gustafson L. Barriers to the Use of Electroconvulsive Therapy in the Elderly: A European Survey. European Psychiatry 17, no.1. 2002.

Pompei P. Delirium in hospitalized elderly patients. Hospitalized elderly patients. Hospital Practice 28: 69, 1993.

Potter WZ, Fink M. How does ECT work? Psychopharmacol Bull 24: 385-386, 1988.

Price TR. Unilateral electroconvulsive therapy for depression (letter) New England Journal of Medicine 304: 53, 1981.

Price TRP, Mc Allister TW. Safety and efficacy of ECT in depressed patients with dementia: a review of clinical experience. Convulsive Therapy 5: 61-74, 1989.

Prinsloo S, Pretorious PJ. Electroconvulsive therapy and its use in modern day psychiatry. South Africa Journal of Psychiatry 10: 38-44, 2004.

Pritchett JT, Kellner CH, Coffey CE. Electroconvulsive therapy in geriatric neuropsychiatry, in Textbook of Geriatric Neuropsychiatry. Edited by Coffey CE, Cummings JL. Washington, DC, American Psychiatric Press, pp 633-660, 1994.

Prudic J, Sackeim HA. Electroconvulsive therapy and the suicide risk. The Journal of Clinical Psychiatry 60 (Suppl): 104-110, 1999.

Quijada SJ. Is ECT Right for You? A Friend to Yourself Resource. 2014.

Rabheru K. Maintence electroconvulsive therapy (M-ECT) after acute response: examining the evidence for who, what, when, and how? Journal of ECT, 28, 39-47, 2012.

Rapinesi C, Kotzalidis GD, Serta D, et al. Prevention of relapse with maintenance electroconvulsive

therapy in elderly patients with major depressive episode. Journal of ECT, 29: 61-64, 2013.

Rajagopal R, Chakrabarti S, Grover S. Satisfation with electroconvulsive therapy among patients and their relatives. Journal of ECT 29: 283-290, 2013.

Rasmussen K, Abrams R. Treatment of Parkinson's Disease with ECT. Psychiatric Clinic North America 14: 925-933, 1991.

Rasmussen KG, Jarvis MR, Zorumski CF. Ketamine anesthesia in electroconvulsive therapy 12: 217-233, 1996.

Ramussen KG. Clinical applications of recent research on electroconvulsive therapy. Bulletin of the Menninger Clinic, Winter vol. 67(1): 18-31, 2003.

Rasmussen KG, Johnson EK, Kung S, et al. An opened-label, pilot study of daily right unilateral ultra brief pulse electroconvulsive therapy. Journal of ECT, 32: 33-37, 2016.

Rasmussen KG, Sampson SM, and Rummans TA. Electroconvulsive Therapy and Newer modalities for the Treatment of Medication-Refractory Mental Illness. Mayo Clinic Proceedings 77, no.6. 2002.

Richardson R, Lowenstein S, Weissberg M. Coping with the suicidal elderly: a physician's guide. Geriatrics 44: 43-51, 1989.

Robinson D, Kubose K, Starr L, et al. Mood changes in stroke patients: relationship to lesion location. Compr Psychiatry 24: 555-566, 1983.

Robinson RG, and Price TR. Post-stroke depressive disorders: A follow-up of 103 patients. Stroke 13: 635-641, 1982.

Rosenberg DR, Wright B, Gershon S. Depression in the elderly. Dementia 3: 157, 1992.

Rudorfer MV and Lebowitz BD. Progress in ECT Research. American Journal of Psychiatry 156, no.6.1999.

Rupke SJ, Blecke D, and Renfrow M. Cognitive therapy for depression. American Family Physician, 73 (1): 83-86, 2006.

Russell JC, Rasmussen KG, O'Conner MK, et al. Long-term maintenance ECT: a retrospective review of

efficacy and cognitive outcome. Journal of ECT 19: 4-9, 2003.

Sackeim HA. Optimizing unilateral electroconvulsive therapy. Convulsive Therapy 7: 201-212, 1991.

Sackeim HA. Devanand DP, and Prudic J. Stimulus Intensity, Seizure Threshold, and Seizure Duration: Impact on the Efficacy and Safety of Electroconvulsive Therapy. Psychiatric Clinics of North America 14, No 4. 1991.

Sackeim HA, Prudic J, Devanand DP, Nobler MS, et al. A Prospective, Randomized, Double-blind Comparison of Bilateral and

Right Unilateral Electroconvulsive Therapy at Different Stimulus Intensities. Archives of General Psychiatry 57, NO. 5. 2000.

Saito S. Anesthesia management for electroconvulsive therapy: hemodynamic and respiratory management. Journal of Anesthesia 19: 142-149, 2005.

Salzman L. An Evaluation of Shock Therapy. American Journal of Psychiatry 103. 1947.

Sackeim HA. Optimizing unilateral electroconvulsive therapy. Convulsive Therapy 7: 201-212. 1991.

Sackeim HA, Decina P, Kanzler M, et al. Effects of electrode placement on the efficacy of titrated, low-dose ECT. American Journal of Psychiatry 144: 1449-1455, 1987.

Sackeim HA, Decina P, Prohovnik I, et al. Seizure threshold in electroconvulsive therapy: effects of sex, age, electrode placement, and number of treatments. Archive General Psychiatry 44: 355-360, 1987.

Sackeim HA, Prudie J, Devanand DP, et al. Effects of stimulus intensity and electrode placement on the efficacy and cognitive effects of electroconvulsive therapy. New England Journal of Medicine 328: 839-846, 1993.

Sackeim HA, Haskett RF, Mulsant BH, et al. Continuation pharmacotherapy in the prevention of relapse following electroconvulsive therapy: a randomized controlled trial. JAMA 285: 1299-1237, 2001.

Sackeim HA, Decina P, Portnoy S, et al. Studies of dosage, seizure threshold, and seizure duration in ECT. Biol Psyciatry. 22: 249-268, 1987.

Sackeim HA, Long J, Luber B, et al. Physical properties and quantification of the ECT stimulus, I: basic principles. Convulsive Therapy 10: 93-123, 1994.

Safferman AZ, Munne R. Combining clozapine with ECT. Case Report. Convulsive Therapy, 8: 141-143, 1992.

Selvin BL. Electroconvulsive therapy-1987. Anesthesiology 67: 367-385, 1987.

Scott AI, Which depressed patients will respond to electroconvulsive therapy? The search for biological predictors of recovery. British Journal of Psychiatry. 154: 81-87, 1989.

Schlogl M, Holick MF. Vitamin D and neurocognitive function. Clinical Interventions in Aging. 9: 559-68, 2014.

Schor JD, Levkoff SE, Lipsitz LA, et al. Risk factors for delirium in hospitalized elderly. JAMA. 267: 827-831, 1992.

Shankel LW, Dimassimo DA, Whittier JR. Changes with age in electrical reactions in mental patients. Psychiatry Questions 34: 284-292, 1960.

Shapira B, Lerer B, Gilboa D, et al. Facilitation of ECT by caffeine pre-treatmetn. American Journal of Psychiatry 144: 1199-1202, 1987.

Shorter E. The History of ECT: Some Unsolved Mysteries. Psychiatric Times 21, No. 2. 2004.

Shorter E and Healy D. Shock Therapy: A history of electroconvulsive treatment in mental illness. Rutgers University Press, 2007.

Sobin. Prudic J, Devanand DP, et al. Who responds to electroconvulsive therapy? A comparison of effective and ineffective forms of treatment. British Journal of Psychiatry 169 322-328, 1996.

Sommer BR, Satlin A, Friedman MS. Glycopyrrolate versus atropine in post-ECT amnesia in the elderly. J Journal of Geriatric Psychiatry Neurol. 2: 18-21, 1989.

Stern L, Dannon PN, Hirschmanns, et al. Aminophylline increases seizure length during electroconvulsive therapy. Journal of ECT. 15:252-257, 1999.

Strain JJ, Brunschwig L, Duffy JP, et al. Comparison of therapeutic effects and memory changes with bilateral and unilateral ECT. American Journal of Psychiatry. 125: 294-304, 1968.

Shapira B, Lerer B, Gilboa D, et al. Facilitation of ECT by caffeine pre-treatment. American Journal of Psychiatry 144: 1199-1202, 1987.

Shapira B, Lere B, Gilboa D, et al. Facilitation of ECT by caffeine pre-treatment. American Journal of Psychiatry. 144: 1199-1202, 1987.

Squire LR. Memory functions as affected by electroconvulsive therapy. Ann NY Acad Sci 462: 307-314, 1986.

Squire LR. Memory functions as affected by electrodes therapy. Ann New York Academy Science 462: 307-314, 1986.

Stromgren LS. Frequency of ECT treatments. Convulsive Therapy 5: 317-318, 1990.

Swartz CM, Larson G. Generalization of the effects of unilateral and bilateral ECT. American Journal of Psychiatry 143: 1040-1041, 1986.

Swartz CM. Anesthesia for ECT. Convulsive Therapy. 9: 301-316, 1993.

Tancer ME, Evans DL. Electroconvulsive therapy in geriatric patients undergoing anticoagulation therapy. Convulsive Therapy. 5:102-9, 1989.

Tanney BL. Electroconvulsive therapy and suicide. Suicide and Life Threatening Behavior, 16: 116-140, 1986.

Taylor JR, Abrams R. Short-term cognitive effects of unilateral and bilateral ECT. British Journal Psychiatry 146: 308-311, 1985.

Thenon J. Electroconvulsive monolateral. Acta Neuropsiquiatria Argentia. 2: 292-296, 1956.

Tueth MJ, Cheong JA. Delirium: diagnosis and treatment in the older patient. Geraitrics 48: 75-80, 1993.

Walling AD. Is it time to reconsider use of ECT for depression? Tips from other Journals. American Family Physician, 2003.

Warnez S, Alessi-Severini S. Clozapine: a review of clinical practice guidelines and prescribing trends. BMC Psychiatry 7: 102, 2014.

Watterson D. The effect of age, head resistance, and other physical factors on the stimulus threshold of electrically induced convulsions. Journal Neurol Neurosurg Psychiatry 8: 121-125, 1945.

Weaver L, Williams R, Rush S. Current density in bilateral and unilateral ECT. Biological Psychiatry 11: 303-312, 1976.

Webb MC, Coffey CE, Saunders WR, et al. Cardiovascular response to unilateral electroconvulsive therapy. Biol Psychiatry 28: 758-768, 1990.

Welch CA, Drop LJ. Cardiovascular effects of ECT. Convulsive Therapy 5: 35-43, 1989.

Wells KB Stewart A, Mays RD, et al. The functioning and well-being of depressed patients. Results from the Medical Outcomes Study. JAMA 262: 914-919, 1989.

Weiner RD. ECT and seizure threshold: effects of stimulus wave form and electrode placement. Biol Psychiatry 15: 225-241, 1980.

Weiner RD, Coffey CE, Krystal AD. The monitoring and management of electrically induced seizures. Psychiatry Clinical North American 14: 845-869, 1991.

Weiner RD, Krystal AD. The present use of electroconvulsive therapy. Annu Rev Med 454: 273-281, 1994.

Weiner RD and Coffey CE. Electroconvulsive Therapy in the United States. Psychopharmacology Bulletin 27, no 1. 1991.

Weiner RD, Coffey CE. Comparison of brief pulse and sine wave stimuli. Convulsive Therapy 5: 184-185, 1989.

Weiner RD, Coffey CE. Comparison of brief-pulse and sine-wave stimuli. Convulsive Therapy 5: 184-185, 1989.

Welch CA, Drop LJ. Cardiovascular effects of ECT. Convulsive Therapy. 5: 35-43, 1989.

Wu CS, Wang SC, Chang IS, Lin KM. The association between dementia and long-term use of benzodiazepine in the elderly: nested case-control study using claims data. The American Journal of Geriatric Psychiatry 17(7): 614-620, 2009.

Yaffe K, Falvey CM, Hoang T. Connections between sleep and cognition in older adults. The Lancet Neurology 13 (10): 1017-28, 2014.

Yesavage JA. Geriatric depression scale. Psychopharm Bull 24: 709-711, 1988.

Zamora EW, Kaelbling R. Memory and electroconvulsive therapy. American Journal of Psychiatry. 122: 546-554, 1965.

Zis AP, Goumeniok AD, Clark CM, et al. ECT-induced prolactin release: effect of sex, electrode placement and serotonin uptake inhibition. Hum Psychopharmacology 6: 155-160, 1991.

Zorumski CF, Burke WJ, Rutherford JL, et al. ECT: Clinical variables, seizure duration, and outcome. Convulsive Therapy. 2: 109-119, 1986.

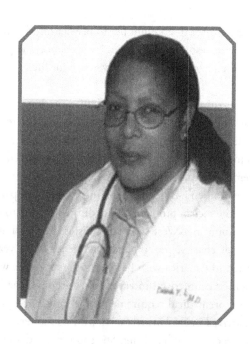

About the Author

Deborah Y. Liggan, M.D. is a physician whose research and writing focus have been to explore the importance of cultural variables in medicine. Her personal biography involves living on three different continents, achieving a varied educational background, and succeeding in both civilian employment and military service. As a young woman, she wanted to be a doctor to generically heal the masses and give ailing bodies the strength to enjoy life. In the years it took her to become eligible for medical school, she met that generic mass. She looked into the swollen face of a burn victim; she rocked the fragile infant who never left the Pediatric Intensive Care Unit; she held the hand of an unwed teen alone in the hour of birth. Most important, she developed caring relationships that taught her to use her mind and heart to achieve the greatest good. Even as a lay spectator, the practice of medicine filled her with awe and reverence for life.

A series of altruistic responses to difficult situations precipitated her pursuit of a medical career. Although she entered college with a solid foundation for the basic sciences and an interest in medicine, she was soon discouraged by the racial tensions and systemic discrimination that followed the desegregation of her private women's college. Resolving to become part of the solution to the racism problem, she dedicated her life to religious service as a nun in a West German cloistered order and upheld rigid vows of chasity, poverty and obedience. Two years later, she returned to America with her commitment to the welfare of others focused on medical intervention. Although she intended to complete premedical requirements and enter medical school, Deborah arrived in the United States with no money, no place to live, and one change of clothing. She soon married and pursued an education while working full-time. Her desire to become a physician conflicted with the traditional marriage her spouse envisioned, and despite compromises and counseling, she was left with a dream and two infant daughters. In the years that followed, Dr. Liggan often worked two jobs to support her family and pay for her education. She completed a Masters of Business Management in 1985 and was commissioned as an officer in the Air Force in 1986. This was an opportunity to provide for the children and become a physician.

Dr. Liggan's motivation to become a physician was the catalyst for her conduct as an officer and community leader. For her professional performance she received distinctions such as Air Training Command Company Grade Officer of the Quarter (1987), Management Effectiveness Inspection Professional Performer (1988), Best of the Best (1988), 432nd Command

Support Group Security Police Officer of the Year (1989), and the Air Force Commendation Medal (1988). Within the community, she led youth activities, managed fund-raising events, and performed volunteer services at the base Emergency Room. Involvement in community activities resulted in her selection as one of the "Four Most Outstanding Blacks" at Misawa Air Base, Japan (1990). Later that year she was selected to participate in the Bridge to Medicine Program at Texas A&M University College of Medicine, followed by matriculation into the 1991 freshman class.

She developed a dissociative model of adolescent substance abuse that received first place accolades in the 1997 Maurice Levine Essay Contest of the Cincinnati Psychiatric Society and was one of the two resident papers selected for presentation at the 1998 Annual Meeting of the American Academy of Psychoanalysis in Ontario, Canada. While she was on active duty, she experienced several episodes with symptoms of elation, depression, insomnia, irritability, confusion, inappropriate flirtatiousness and dating, delusional thinking, and suicidal preoccupation and attempts. Dr. Liggan stated in her psychiatric interview that she was angry at being hospitalized and felt like a failure in that she had not killed herself. She attempted suicide twice, once by hanging and again by overdose of 250 Ibuprofen. She received ten ECT treatments which improved her mood and decreased her hopelessness and suicidal ideas. This was followed by a total of 270 maintenance ECT treatments over 15 years. All treatments were administered with bilateral electrode placement using constant current, brief-pulse ECT devices. Dr. Liggan is now on a medical retirement form the Air Force based on a Bipolar Disorder with Psychotic Features.

To highlight the importance of cultural variables in psychotherapy, Dr. Liggan explored the literature on racial issues in the dynamic psychotherapy of African Americans. This resulted in a paper that was awarded the 1997 John Spiegel Fellowship by the Society for the Study of Psychiatry and Culture, as well as publications in the journal Transcultural Psychiatry. Her exploration of cultural variables in medical diagnoses began with a look at ectopic pregnancy in African American females, which was published in Minority Health Today.

In 2009 she published "Taking Care of Our Folks" which draws on comprehensive and detailed research to ensure that elderly African-Americans receive culturally competent healthcare and live more productive, independent, and pain-free lives. Because of this growing population, taking care of elderly patients has become the responsibility of their family.

In 2015 she published "The Veteran's Guide to Psychiatry" which continues to play a central role in providing mental health services by caring for those who served our country. Topics focus specifically on veterans and include psychiatric interviewing, mood disorders, anxiety disorders, psychotic disorders, disorders of cognition, recovery from mental illness, and psychiatric emergencies.

INDEX

B

C

Mental Status Examination, 27-31
Methohexital, 31,46, 164
Metrazol Therapy, 17, 160
Meyer, Adolf, 97, 101
Monoamine Oxidase Inhibitors (MAOIs), 39, 119-120
Mouthguard, 33, 42, 49, 53, 67, 179
Muscle relaxant, 3, 49, 66-67, 161, 169
Myocardinal infarction, 145- 146

N

National Alliance on Mental Illness, 80
Nausea, 62-63, 166
Neurobiologic features, 75-78
Neuroleptic Malignant Syndrome
Neuro-muscular blocking agents, 76
Neurosyphilis, 13
Neurotransmitter Therapy, 17-18
Neurovegetative Functions, 66, 167, 170
Niacin
Nocturnal myoclonus, 109, 122, 174
Nonsteroidal anti-inflammatory drugs (NSAIDs)
Noradrenergic function
Norepinephrine, 118

Normal Pressure Hydrocephalus, 134
Nutrition, 17-18, 43

O

Obsessive-Compulsive Disorder, 175
Orthostatic hypotension, 175
Osteoporosis, 5, 158
Ottosson, JO, 4
Outpatient ECT, 7
Oxygen
Oxygenation, 3, 19, 165

P

Paranoid Personality, 101
Parkinson's Disease, 134-135, 180
Parisian Asylum Psychiatrists
• Pascal, Constance, 13-14
Pavlov, Ivan, 97
Pellagra
Penicillin
Personality disorders, 112, 176
Petit mal Seizures, 143
Pharmacokinetics
Pick's Disease, 132
Pneumonia, 149
Postictal care, 57-63, 159
Post-stroke depression
Post-Traumatic Stress Disorder (PTSD)
Pre-ECT Evaluation, 25-26, 32-33

Printed in the United States
By Bookmasters